SAGE

BREASTFEEDING

Nourished and Connected

Rachel Rainbolt, M.A., CEIM

The Sage Parenting Series

1. Sage Parenting: Honored and Connected
2. Sage Sleep: Rested and Connected
3. Sage Breastfeeding: Nourished and Connected
4. Sage Homeschooling: Wise and Connected

Written by Rachel Rainbolt, M.A., CEIM
Edited by Casey Ebert, M.F.A.

Disclaimer

I recommend that parents consider options and become as informed as is possible, matching what you learn with what you think can work the best for your child(ren), you, and your family. You must use your wisdom and discretion in deciding what is in the best interest of your child(ren). The material in this book is meant to be considered in this process, providing relevant information, perspective, anecdotes, tools, and techniques for your inspiration and consideration. The products and product considerations recommended in this book are personal preferences. You are encouraged to investigate and form your own opinions as to the rightness of fit of any product for your child and you. The information in this book is not meant to be considered medical or psychotherapeutic advice. Rachel Rainbolt, Sage Parenting, is not liable or responsible for the parenting choices you make, actions you take, or any consequences thereof.

DEDICATION

Thank you to my mother for breastfeeding me against so many odds. You nurtured me.

Thank you to my sister for role modeling the normal way to feed babies. You taught me.

Thank you to my college classmate for sharing your personal breastfeeding photos from around the world for a project. You inspired me.

Thank you to my husband for always bringing me water and standing by my side proudly for every effort of breastfeeding advocacy. You support me.

Thank you to my three nurslings for being the wisest half of our breastfeeding relationship. You shape me.

CONTENTS

1

BREASTFEEDING MY WEST

Breastfeeding is how my baby and I plug into each other, creating a connection through which his body, mind, heart, and soul are all fed. If he is hungry, our connection provides him sustenance. If he is tired, our connection lulls him. If he is distressed, our connection soothes him. If he is discomforted, our connection eases the discomfort. If he is ill, our connection is all the medicine he needs. If he is overstimulated, the rest of the world fades away and disappears as he becomes lost in our connection. If he is joyful, our connection sets the stage for the dance of interaction between our faces.

It is spiritual. It is practical. It is so much between my baby and me. It is a physical experience to complement, reflect, and facilitate a magnificent bond. To be able to experience such a physical reaction to his cry, with the letdown of milk and the physical discomfort of being swollen with longing from the engorgement that follows separation, is relieving and cathartic, providing a physical outlet for so much that exists between us. I give and he receives, but without his interactive presence and need, I would have nothing to give. It requires of us both, and from it we reap rewards that transcend what anyone else can see and what can be read on a list of benefits.

As he latches, a true and total peace washes over his face. In that moment and those that follow, he wants for nothing, his every need met. The moments preceding are forgotten, and no experience outside the current exchange between us matters or even seems to have ever mattered. Our breastfeeding time together forces me to carve out a sanctuary for the two of us, insulated from the agenda of the day and the demands of life. Here in this cloud we float together, warm and cozy, insulated from the storms of the world.

From any pain, challenges, or obstacles spring only elevated devotion, dedication, and investment in this harborer of my love returned to me, my future. You are worth every ounce of this miraculous part of me I give to you: this gift of breastmilk.

2

BREASTFEEDING ON CUE

At your first pediatric appointment with your new baby you are always asked, "How often do you feed them?" This question may seem innocuous to the unsuspecting new parent, but beware! It is a loaded question. The conversation with me goes something like this:

"How often do you feed him?"

"Whenever he wants to breastfeed."

"How often is that?"

"However often he wants to breastfeed."

"Are you feeding him every two hours?"

"No. I am feeding him whenever he wants to breastfeed."

"Well, we need to know, so you need to keep track."

"No, actually, I don't. We both need to know if he is healthy and thriving, and I invite you to observe my healthy, thriving baby. And he got this way by being breastfed on cue and not on a schedule. I base my parenting decisions on what is in the best interest of my baby, not what makes it most convenient for you to fill out your chart."

Cue disgruntled nurse exiting exam room. Could I be called a bitch? Perhaps, but I am 100% okay with being disliked for standing up for what I know is in the best interest of my baby. A lot of moms would just say, "Sure, every two hours." You pick and choose your battles, and this is a battle I choose because that question doesn't just ask you for information, it tells you that you should be scheduling your infant's feedings. This question leaves the mom, who has been following her maternal wisdom, responding sensitively to her baby's cues, and feeding them when they want to breastfeed, thinking: "Oh my goodness. I'm supposed to know how often he breastfeeds? Why don't I know how often he breastfeeds? I'm supposed to feed him every two hours? Oh my goodness. This is how all moms feed their babies? If the nurse is implying that I should be breastfeeding him on a schedule, then that must be what is healthiest for him."

> Tip: If you choose to vaccinate your baby, consider having the nurse administer the shots while your baby is breastfeeding in your arms. Much of the distress and trauma babies communicate in their panicked cry during immunizations is more from being removed from the safe harbor of Mommy's arms and pinned to a table by strangers. Hold and breastfeed your baby, lovingly hold their leg with your free hand, and the nurse can quickly administer their shot(s). From the security of your embrace and with the oxytocin (the euphoria-inducing bonding hormone) high of nursing, your baby may barely even notice the poke and be quickly lulled back to contentment.

Brain-Body Connection

Babies are born knowing few things; if nothing else, they have an amazingly strong mind-body connection—they know how to listen to their bodies. This means that they eat when they are hungry. They sleep when they are tired. They seek comfort when they need it. You cannot over-breastfeed a baby. If you foster this mind-body connection, you encourage your child to listen to the signals of their body and allow those to guide them (Breastmilk actually contains a hormone called Leptin, which, after being received in the first months of breastfeeding on cue, provides the physiological foundation for food intake regulation for the long haul.[82]). Fast forward and this looks like a child who eats when they are hungry and stops when they are no longer hungry. If you interrupt this connection in an attempt to seize control of your baby's feedings, you teach your child to ignore the signals of their body. "Eat when there is food in front of you. Eat until it is gone because you won't be able to eat again, even if you are hungry." Eating is about a schedule. Eating becomes more about the power struggle between parent and child and not about satisfying needs. Furthermore, there is a loss of trust between parent and infant when an infant reaches out, communicates that they have a need, and that need is not met.

Supply and Demand

In addition to the mind-body connection within your baby, there is an amazing breast-baby connection that flourishes when you breastfeed on cue. Your milk supply will perfectly attune to your baby's ever-changing nutritional needs. If your baby is having a growth spurt and needs more milk, as long as you offer it (put them to breast whenever they are hungry), your milk supply will increase to perfectly meet their need. With only a 24-hour layover time, your breasts will adjust to every change in their natural routine, ensuring their every need is met. All you have to do to allow this perfectly honed system to function is breastfeed on cue.

Motivation

Breastfeeding according to the cues of your baby meets needs that you may not even be aware of. Did you know that your nipple absorbs your baby's saliva, reads the germ content, and tailors the milk with antibodies to combat the particular illnesses to which your baby has been exposed? Your baby may want to breastfeed what seems like constantly for days and emerge from this period as though nothing ever happened. They could have been fighting an illness that your breastmilk defeated. They may have been loading up for a growth spurt. The beauty of the system is that you and your baby don't even have to be aware of the motives at play. You just have to trust the system. "Ground breaking lactation research demonstrates that there is an intricate method of communication in the saliva of a baby that triggers mother's milk production via receptors on the areola. This communication signals all of baby's needs to mother by way of hormones and enzymes (and likely things we have not even begun to understand). How much milk your baby needs, the fat/calories composition he requires today, what specific antibodies he needs a boost of, the immunological properties he requires most right now—it is all transferred to you and your body's amazing milk making wisdom via your baby's sucking at your breast."[1]

Trusting the System

I received a plea from a new-mama friend asking for any advice on boosting milk supply before she switched to half formula supplementation for her 4-week-old. My reflexive response was to ask how often she was breastfeeding. "One to two times a day." Why? Her nipples were sore, she wanted to let Daddy feed Baby, she wanted to know how much milk Baby was getting at each feeding to make sure he was getting enough, and they were sleep training at night.

Mother Nature delivers a baby to your chest naked, skin-to-skin, with no baggage. There is nothing between you and your baby. You need only surrender to Baby's needs as a guide and you will be on the right path. Then, out of a well-intentioned drive to do everything "right," we promptly cram a heap of shit between our babies and ourselves. Ironically, this is the very point at which we go wrong, veering off the path and becoming our own worst enemies.

My response? "Okay, lots of stumbling blocks in that one sentence . . ." and I proceeded to dismantle those Booby Traps[33] one by one. Don't assume something that has worked for millions of years is suddenly not working. Success is the norm. *Lean in* to breastfeeding and trust the system.

Another friend was frantically searching for honey to put on her 4-week-old's pacifier after he was accidentally hurt (note: never give honey to a baby younger than 12 months old, as it can contain botulism spores that act as a neurotoxin in an infant's digestive system[29]). I warned her of the danger of honey for infants (she was unaware), and she asked if I had any other suggestions. I suggested breastfeeding him, which was dismissed out of hand because, "The pediatrician said I should not be feeding him more than once every two hours. Plus, he's not hungry." "I can see that hearing him cry is causing a physical reaction in you. What are you feeling? What do you think he is telling you he needs? What is your body compelling you to do? What is your maternal wisdom suggesting?"

You don't need permission to breastfeed your baby on cue. You don't need my approval, your pediatrician's, or your mother's to meet your baby's needs. Respond sensitively and consistently. Listen to your baby and honor your maternal wisdom. Nurse without fear whenever your baby gives you a cue. It is in their best interest, and yours.

Night Nursing

Breastfeeding on cue is particularly valuable after sunset. Breastmilk production actually increases at nighttime (thanks to nightly piqued Prolactin levels (the milk producing hormone)) to facilitate night nursing because breastmilk that is produced at night actually contains melatonin, a sleep-inducing hormone that infants do not produce on their own, as well as a sleep-inducing amino acid called tryptophan. Melatonin is a magical substance, which is present in adults and undetectable in infants, that induces sleep (among other numerous positive benefits). Melatonin is found in the breastmilk produced by Mom at bedtime and during the night. It is not in formula and it is not in breastmilk produced during the day. Studies show that babies who are breastfed on cue during the evening and night cry less, have eased digestive systems, and *sleep more*. When your baby attempts to cluster feed (nurse on and off for a long stretch of time) for that last nursing session of the night before their first and longest stretch of sleep, they are flooding their system with melatonin, which shifts their body into sleep mode.[18] To learn everything you need to know to have harmoniously restful nights with your baby, read my book *Sage Sleep: Rested and Connected*.[48]

Cues

What are these "cues" we speak of? Every baby is different, and your most valuable asset is going to be to get to know your particular little one, who will have their own unique style of communication. In the beginning, to get to know the language of your baby, it's simplest just to offer the breast any time your baby is not content. It's easy to offer. Keep in mind we are looking for subtle cues. Ideally we want to respond during the pre-cry communication window. (To learn all about crying, read the Cry Baby chapter in my *Sage Parenting* book.[19])

Sometimes it will ease the discontent and meet the need. Sometimes it won't. Sometimes your baby will want to nurse. Sometimes your baby won't. But in offering something that does meet the vast majority of an infant's needs (in response to hunger, discomfort, over-stimulation, tiredness, etc.), you are greatly stacking the cards in your favor for a successful interaction, drawing you together and enhancing your bond. And each time you witness a cue, offer, and see the result, you are becoming more of an expert in the cues of your baby.

Positioning

I owned a breastfeeding pillow, but it didn't rule my breastfeeding sessions; I spent most of my breastfeeding time at home just being comfortable. That was the technical breastfeeding position I employed: comfort. Upright breastfeeding positions, even with a special pillow, might be helpful for some (for example, if you are struggling with a latch), but in order for me to be content and happy breastfeeding on cue for hours at a time, I needed comfort that these positions did not provide. I would deeply recline on my sofa and my baby would lie on top of me, parallel to my body, belly to belly. Sometimes I would shove a pillow under one arm. I would have the end table next to me stashed with water, a snack, my phone to communicate with the outside world, my laptop to do work, an iPad to read books, or the remote to watch TV. You can achieve the same effect in your bed with pillows for propping you up at just the right angle. Were I sitting upright with my feet on the floor in a wooden rocking chair with a baby perpendicular across my chest, my nursing sessions would have been significantly shortened. Imagine my surprise when I discovered that my breastfeeding style was an actual movement or school of thought in the lactation consulting world referred to as Biological Nurturing.[41] I didn't know this was a special style of breastfeeding; I thought it was just . . . breastfeeding. After all, newborns are designed with that stepping reflex to crawl up your front and latch onto your nipple (the breast crawl). I feel like Mother Nature intended this more intuitive style of nursing. The takeaway here is that to truly embrace breastfeeding on cue you should nurse in positions that are comfortable for you. Your baby might breastfeed for 10 minutes or for two hours. If it's not working for you, it's not going to work.

Altogether

I find that the more we can simplify, the more successful parents can be and the better the relationship between baby and parent. When you can bulldoze aside concerns such as following schedules, trying to ascertain a singular "true" motive behind a breastfeeding request ("Is she really hungry?"), fearing behavioral ramifications of meeting an infant's needs (you can*not* spoil a baby), nursing in the "right" position, etc., what is left is the beautiful simplicity of you and your baby. Your loving attachment is given the silence and space it needs to be the loudest presence in your mind. These are the conditions under which breastfeeding can lay the foundation for a rewarding, intuitive, lifelong bond.

Luckily for parents and infants, breastfeeding meets many needs for a baby. This makes the system of cue and response pretty simple. My baby West, who would breastfeed as I typed, would be lying on me when his arms and legs would begin to move more abruptly. He would turn his face to the side (grunting and slobbering), slightly raising the right side of his upper lip. My milk would let down as I pulled aside my shirt, and he would latch and breastfeed for about 10 minutes, fall asleep, and then roll his head onto the center of my chest. Was he hungry? Yes. Was he tired? Yes. Was he in need of some intimate bonding time? Yes. Mission accomplished on all fronts. It is such a perfect system, such a beautiful dance that takes place between us, and as long as we move to the rhythm, we are in sync, in perfect harmony. Whether I am doing some email coaching or on a hike with my kids, I cannot imagine a more convenient and healthy life for my baby and me. I trust him and he trusts me. What an amazing foundation for a loving relationship.

3

NURSING IN PUBLIC

Breastfeeding in public is just breastfeeding. You live one life, in one world that belongs to all of us. It is not possible to designate breastfeeding as a private activity because it is not possible to live a life exclusively in private. Embrace breastfeeding on cue and live your life out in the world.

The Practical

Babymoon

The first few weeks of breastfeeding can be hard. The cocooned state of the babymoon lends itself perfectly to giving you the comfortable space you need to get your breastfeeding footing and work through any potentially painful challenges that can mark the first weeks of your breastfeeding journey. It takes practice and guidance to successfully exit your babymoon with breasts and a baby who respond to each other with ease. But once you are over the hump, life is sweet. This is when you are ready to leave the safety net of your breastfeeding nest and step excitedly into the current of society as your baby's mommy.

On Cue

Feeding on cue is the perfect way to have a successful, easy, convenient breastfeeding relationship, even and especially in public. Trying to schedule your baby's feeding sessions puts a lot of pressure on you and a mountain of pressure on your baby. You are really setting yourself up for failure if you simultaneously limit your access to the world and deny your baby their coping mechanism by restricting your breastfeeding to a schedule. Breastfeeding on cue means you have everything and exactly what Baby needs, in every situation and at all times. Your baby is "society friendly," contentedly willing to go anywhere and tolerate most anything as long as they have their mommy milk at hand.

Babywearing

Breastfeeding in public comes together with babywearing in perfect harmony to give you access to all society has to offer. Once you master breastfeeding in a sling, wrap, or carrier, the world is your oyster. You no longer even require a place to sit or two free hands. I can breastfeed my baby while pushing a shopping cart and holding my older son's hand in the grocery store, all with comfort and discretion.

Attempting to nurse while babywearing for the first time while you are out in the world, feeling the pressure of the current around you and the stress of a hungry baby, is a recipe for failure. Begin by breastfeeding at home, outside of the pouch, in the position Baby will nurse in inside the pouch. For example, if you are nursing in a soft, structured carrier, Baby will be sitting in your lap facing you, looking out to the side while you support your breast from the outside. After you get comfortable here, practice breastfeeding in the pouch at home in front of a mirror, then while walking around the house, then while out on a walk, then out in the world (I have some You Tube videos that can help with this[77]). In no time you will be a babywearing-breastfeeding pro, ready to conquer the world.

Clothing

I find that it is helpful and worth the investment to buy some shirts that easily facilitate breastfeeding in public. You can also go through your existing wardrobe with a fresh pair of eyes, looking at your clothes from a new perspective with the priority of boob access. A set of camisole tank tops with an elastic neckline can be worn under any shirt that can easily be lifted to create a comfortable and discreet nursing setup. Any time your baby wants to nurse, you simply reach under the over shirt, lower the cami tank and raise the over shirt just enough to latch baby. This is a beautiful setup because your baby has access, your breast is covered, your belly is covered, and you can still see your baby's face. If you are breastfeeding in a sling or carrier, I highly recommend shirts that either have a neckline that stretches below your breast or button down from the top. While wearing your baby in a sling, it is difficult to pull a shirt up but easy to lower or unbutton a shirt from the top down, and the sling or carrier provides any privacy you may want. I also recommend investing in some good nursing bras. They can keep you comfortable and supported and provide convenient access for breastfeeding out in the world.

Cover

I don't use a breastfeeding cover. Some moms do. If you find it helpful to your breastfeeding success, then use it. If you don't, then don't. Be sure to respect your baby's needs and comfort along with yours in making the decision. And be open to trying a variety of setups to find what feels right for you and your little one. For example, a scarf can be both fashionable and helpful in covering any exposed breast flesh that causes you discomfort while leaving your baby's head and face out in the fresh air. I find that breastfeeding in the pouch provides ample discretion. The most important takeaway here is that it is your decision and yours alone. The pressure or insistence that a woman covers more or less is oppressive. I support you, in whatever makes you comfortable. Period.

Peep Show or Parenting?

In addition to the practical preparation and skills, it is, unfortunately, necessary in this present society to address the social stigma associated with breastfeeding in public. Some psychological shoring up can go a long way in preparing you to exude confidence as a badass breastfeeder.[26]

Role Modeling

The only reason breastfeeding makes some onlookers uncomfortable is that it is sadly too rare a sight. *Breastfeeding in public normalizes breastfeeding.* Merely by doing what is normal and healthy in the course of your everyday life, you encourage other women to breastfeed, model how it is done, and socialize support. If children grow up and people everywhere live their lives seeing breastfeeding, it becomes simply how a baby eats: the mundane, everyday act of feeding a baby.

History

The social stigma surrounding breastfeeding in public is very recent. Throughout the course of human history, across virtually every culture around the world, breastfeeding was universally accepted without condition (as it would need to be for a society to survive). The Virgin Mary and Jesus did it (and were later even honored in prominent artwork[27] doing so— the viral pic of its Renaissance time). The prude

Puritans, covered from neck to toe, felt it commonplace to pull out a breast and feed a hungry baby in the town square (shock—"whipping it out" sans hooter hider!). Those stoic Victorians even prided themselves on their creepy, gaunt-faced breastfeeding portraits[28] (holla, badass, ghost-like breastfeeding mamas!).

Breastfeeding in public enjoyed a good all-of-human-existence-long run until the advent of formula and the bottle, which is very recent in human history. (Now before you get your panties in a twist with defensive outrage, I am not demonizing any formula-feeding or bottle-using mommies. This is a sociological history lesson to contextualize how we ended up here so we can be informed and empowered in moving forward.) Formula companies, faced with marketing their product in the time of the Great Depression (an alternative for a substance that was FREE), successfully crafted a product identity rooted in status. It was a product for babies whose families could afford it. It worked. Breastfeeding became associated with the lower class. Once breastfeeding was no longer seen on a regular basis, it was no longer the norm and was soon shrouded in shame.

Now that valid scientific research has unequivocally emphasized the importance of breastfeeding for a healthy population, efforts have been made to encourage mothers to breastfeed. As breastfeeding rates have risen due to this education aimed directly at mothers, societal acceptance and support of the practical side of breastfeeding have lagged. We now know that "breast is best," and society is quick to tell you this but slow to show you in the form of unconditional acceptance and support. We're left in a no man's land of "you should breastfeed" but . . . "you shouldn't breastfeed." We can't have it both ways! It sets mothers up to fail (and by "fail" I mean fail to meet their breastfeeding goals, whatever they may be) when we don't support breastfeeding mothers in action. Breastfeeding in public is where the rubber meets the road.

Social Media

Social media has fortunately become a monumentally huge platform for breastfeeding support as mothers are being instantly connected with thousands of other women in support of all their breastfeeding struggles and triumphs.[49] You can tap into this support by simply following pages and joining groups that resonate with your experience and perspective, and engaging. On your own pages, feel free to share the photos and experiences that make up your mothering journey, which is so much of your life and who you are in this season. This includes breastfeeding, which occupies a significant amount of your time and focus. Wondering if you should post that photo or anecdote? Would you hesitate if there were a bottle instead of a breast? No? Then post it. If your social media pages are to be an authentic representation of you, then you should not feel the need to banish breastfeeding as a shameful secret (let your super boobies come out of the closet). You should feel comfortable celebrating all that makes you the amazing mama you are, including breastfeeding. And remember: breastfeeding in public normalizes breastfeeding. This applies to the virtual world just as to the real one. Also know that there are no social media sites I have ever been on that classify breastfeeding photos as indecent, as the act of breastfeeding is *not* indecent.

My only word of caution is to beware the trolls. As we all know, there is an online phenomenon of commenters sitting around all day and night trying to virtually (and cruelly) poke everyone with a sharp stick. Ignore them. It is a symptom of an exchange where people remain faceless, where the weak and hurt allow their ids to drive and they do not receive the consequence of the face-to-face feedback of their victims. The cardinal rule of trolling is "Don't feed the trolls." They don't mean what they say and they will not consider your thoughtful response.

16 Responses to Nursing in Public Idiocy

While discrimination against breastfeeding in public is completely without merit, there are a few ignorant arguments that have been repeated so often they warrant addressing. So let's get a few things straight:

1. If you can expose your breasts in public, then can I expose my penis in public?

Breasts are not sexual organs. Breasts are not part of the female reproductive system. Breasts are not comparable to a penis. Unless you're ready to accept dildos as freely and openly in public as a bottle, don't make this comparison. Exposing a vulva in public would be an appropriate comparison to exposing a penis.

Breasts are secondary sex characteristics, just like other indicators of sex (meaning male versus female) in the species such as height, facial hair, Adam's apple, etc.—none of which are sexual or inappropriate in public.

2. Breasts are used during sex, therefore not appropriate in public.

Breasts are erogenous zones that can be used for sexual arousal just like mouths, fingers, necks, etc. It is acceptable to use your mouth to eat in public, as that is its primary function. It is acceptable to breastfeed in public, as that is your breasts' primary function.

3. Everyone thinks breastfeeding in public is inappropriate.

Just the fact that many people believe something to be so does not make it so. The cultural argument that we should accept the inappropriateness of breastfeeding as objective fact because many people in our society believe it to be so is no truer for breastfeeding discrimination than for segregation by race. It is not okay to try to force people to move to the back of the bus because of their race or a biological function of their sex. We can stand up to misinformed beliefs that do not serve the well-being of our society and those beliefs can change.

4. Be considerate of the fact that you are making others uncomfortable.

Potential discomfort/arousal/offense of someone else is neither my baby's problem nor my responsibility. I don't consider the potential arousal of lurking foot-fetish perverts when I choose my shoes in the morning. Furthermore, we don't get the right to never be uncomfortable or offended. Ignorance offends me and makes me uncomfortable, yet ignorant people still exist. So, if breastfeeding makes people uncomfortable, they are welcome to eat their lunch in the bathroom or eat with a blanket over their head. If people have a problem with breastfeeding, it is their problem, not yours, and certainly not your baby's. *My baby's right to eat trumps your nonexistent right to never see something that makes you uncomfortable.*

5. Peeing is natural too.

Peeing and pooping in public are illegal because they expose genitals and are unsanitary—breastfeeding does/is neither. Breastmilk is food, while urine is human waste that is hazardous to health if expelled in public places.

6. Can't you just pump and feed your baby a bottle while you're out in public?

While some moms can pump and bottle-feed their babies breastmilk in public, it is not possible/advisable/practical for most. You could grocery shop, cook, eat, and clean up your lunch in the privacy of your own home if you'd rather not see me breastfeeding in this restaurant.

A. Pumping and bottle-feeding requires owning a pump, milk storage containers, bottles, artificial nipples, temperature control storage bags, sterilizers, etc. I own none of these things. That's part of the wonderfulness of breastfeeding—it's free.

B. A pump will not trigger the letdown reflex that releases milk in every woman (myself included).

C. Not every baby will take a bottle (my babe has never even seen one).

D. Sometimes a baby will eat five times over the course of half an hour. Sometimes a baby will eat once in five hours. You cannot effectively meet these ever changing feeding needs on cue with supplies prepared and packed in advance. If a baby wants to eat five times and you have one bottle of stored milk, Baby is starving. If you have five bottles of milk and baby eats once, all of that made, pumped, and stored milk is completely wasted ("and leaves you dumping the wasted milk down the sink, screaming 'NO!!!!' on the inside and feeling like those moments in movies when rich people start burning hundred dollar bills."[2]).

E. If your baby is hungry and being fed with a bottle, then you must pump at that same time to maintain your supply. Meaning, instead of breastfeeding your baby in the restaurant booth, you need to use a breast pump in the restaurant booth. Is that really less conspicuous?

F. Bottles of breastmilk must be heated before

given to a baby. When out in the world, there is not usually a way to do this.

G. Much of the benefit of breastfeeding comes from the actual act of breastfeeding. Putting Baby directly on the tap has a myriad of benefits not captured with bottle-feeding. For example (as discussed in Chapter 5), did you know that your areola absorbs your baby's saliva, reads the germ content, and tailors the antibodies in your milk specifically to the germs your baby has been exposed to? That milk magic doesn't happen with a pump and bottle.

7. He's too old to be doing that (if he can ask for it, eat "real" food, has teeth, can walk up to it, etc.).

The age and/or ability of my little one to speak, consume solid food, sprout teeth, stand, or any other arbitrary developmental milestone have no bearing on the appropriateness of breastfeeding in public. The long-lived benefits to breastfeeding extend well beyond infancy (the World Health Organization (WHO) recommends breastfeeding for 2 years and beyond as is mutually desired by mother and baby, with a worldwide average age of weaning around 4), and the weaning of my child is a transition with two people who matter: mother and baby. If you are neither, it is none of your business.

8. There are children here!

Children are always exposed to breastfeeding as the act requires the participation of a child. Furthermore, underage witnesses to the normal process of feeding a baby naturally only serve to normalize breastfeeding for generations to come. Just to be on the safe side, I will provide you with a script to handle the awkward, complicated, in depth conversation that could arise when a child witnesses a baby being fed for the first time:

"What's she doing?"

"Feeding her baby."

Extra material for an older or especially inquisitive child, who is in turn more vulnerable to the dangers of exposure to breastfeeding:
"Babies drink milk from their mommies' breasts."

9. You need to cover up!

Some women choose to breastfeed with a cover for a variety of reasons. Some do not. You know who gets to decide whether or not she uses a cover? Not you. The assertion that any woman should cover more or less is oppressive.

If seeing me breastfeed makes you uncomfortable, you are welcome to eat with a blanket over your head. That is no more absurd than expecting my baby to eat with a blanket over his head.

    A. It gets very hot with your face under a blanket while on someone's chest. I am not willing to suffocate or overheat my baby for your comfort.

    B. Wrestling with a blanket or cover creates a whole other obstacle in the breastfeeding process. Mastering latching a wiggling, hungry baby to your leaking nipple is hard enough without blocking your view and having to keep a piece of fabric draped and secured around you.

C. It's one more piece of bulky gear that I won't lug around with me everywhere I go.

D. Not many babies will tolerate having a sheet held over their faces. My baby would immediately start screaming and flailing in a panic (I can't say I blame him), which is far more socially disruptive than a quiet, calm, silent, content, nursing baby.

10. Be modest and classy.

A woman's willingness to feed her child is in no way an indication of a lack of class or modesty. Even Pope Francis said, "If they are hungry, mothers, feed them, without thinking twice," while encouraging moms to breastfeed uncovered, in public, and on cue.[72] If your standards for class and modesty are more conservative than the Catholic Pope's, they need to be adjusted.

11. Why are women suddenly breastfeeding in public? Our mothers breastfed in private.

Women are not suddenly breastfeeding in public. Human infants have been breastfed in public since the dawn of humanity, otherwise our species would have long ago died out. Women, even during incredibly "modesty" and "purity" focused times, breastfed in public. You know what else they did? Celebrated it by taking breastfeeding photos and commissioning breastfeeding artwork (the social media pic of its day, remember). Also, statistically speaking, our mothers didn't breastfeed. That's why you didn't grow up seeing breastfeeding throughout the course of normal life in society. Thankfully, the tide is again shifting back to breastfeeding as the normal way to feed a baby. And since mothers live life just like you do—out in the world—breastfeeding in public is a part of the new norm.

12. Go do that in the bathroom.

The notion of a baby eating on a public toilet is horrifying. It is no more sanitary for a baby to eat on a public toilet than it would be for you to eat your lunch sitting on a public toilet in a bathroom stall. Actually, as your adult immune system is much stronger than a baby's, it would be more appropriate for you to eat in the bathroom if you are uncomfortable.

13. That's illegal.

Actually, breastfeeding in public is a legally protected right. Furthermore, breastfeeding discrimination, which is sex discrimination based on a biological function of being a woman, is illegal.

In California, Cal. Civ. Code 43.3 (1997) states: "Notwithstanding any other provision of law, a mother may breastfeed her child in any location, public or private, except the private home or residence of another, where the mother and the child are otherwise authorized to be present." Meaning, a woman has the right to breastfeed anywhere she and her baby are allowed to be. Furthermore, the CA Unruh Civil Rights Act specifically covers breastfeeding discrimination as a sex discrimination case.

14. You're only sharing breastfeeding photos to get attention.

    A. Parents are sharing breastfeeding photos because breastfeeding is a significant part of life with a little one. As such, women are capturing photos and documenting experiences around breastfeeding along with all those staples of parenthood like angelic sleeping baby faces and messy eating adventures. They share these photos in the exact same vein as all normal mothering experiences. When you devote a lot of time, energy, and heart to something, you want to share it.

    B. Breastfeeding in public normalizes breastfeeding. Or as my friend Baby's Breastie[1] points out, breastfeeding in public normalizes society, as breastfeeding itself is already the biological norm. This applies to the virtual world just as to the real one.

    C. There are no social media sites that classify breastfeeding photos as indecent, as the act of breastfeeding is not indecent.

15. Breastfeeding a kid like that is psychosexually damaging.

The biological function of breasts is to feed children. In fact, a defining characteristic of mammality is the act of breastfeeding. As breastfeeding is the evolutionary standard, measures of psychosexual health would be based on the species norm, which is to breastfeed for a few years (until we lose our "milk teeth"). So we look at the potentially damaging effects of deviating from the biological norm on healthy psychosexual development: Are there psychosexually damaging effects for children who are prematurely weaned? What are the long-term psychosexual consequences for a person who is prematurely weaning from breastfeeding?

16. I support breastfeeding but . . .

No buts; either you support breastfeeding or you do not. Period.
A good rule of thumb is: if it would be appropriate to feed a baby a bottle in the present setting, then it would be appropriate to breastfeed a baby.

Say What?

Every breastfeeding mother should know and be confident in asserting her legal right to breastfeed in public anywhere she and her baby are allowed to be. Most people are kind, considerate, and supportive. You may well go your entire breastfeeding journey encountering nothing but positive interactions. However, there are some ignorant people in our society whom you could, unfortunately, encounter. I encourage you so vehemently not to give anyone else the power to take away your freedom (making you feel like you shouldn't ever leave your home) or your contentment and pride.

I have breastfed three children, and it was all magic and unicorns until my third nursling was over a year old. That is seven years of breastfeeding in public with only peace before I was slapped in the face with breastfeeding discrimination. You can read about my journey standing my ground and fighting for enforcement of the law protecting a woman's right to breastfeed (and a baby's right to eat) in my article: "Nursing in Public Discrimination: My Journey."[21]

Legal

Laws vary from state to state, so be familiar with the verbiage where you live. As previously mentioned, in California, Cal. Civ. Code 43.3 (1997) states: "Notwithstanding any other provision of law, a mother may breastfeed her child in any location, public or private, except the private home or residence of another, where the mother and the child are otherwise authorized to be present."[32]

Response

If you ever encounter an unsupportive or discriminatory person in the face of your breastfeeding in public journey, maintaining a *calm* yet *confident* state of mind is the foundation of a successful response. This is the most difficult step in the process as the sense of shock and feeling of shame can be overwhelming. Know that there is an entire community of passionate breastfeeding mamas standing right behind you supporting you.

After checking in with yourself to center your

emotional state, reflect back what the person is really saying as a question. This serves as a mirror for the person (reflecting back the direct meaning at the core of their message) and buys you an extra couple of minutes to get your bearings. "Are you telling me that I cannot breastfeed in your business?"

The next step is to educate the individual on the law. "Breastfeeding in public is actually a legally protected right. I have the right to breastfeed my baby anywhere my baby and I are allowed to be, with no conditions."

This is where the situation can go one of two ways: either the person backs down and leaves you in peace or they irrationally push forward. "Well, I'm going to need you to stop/cover/do that in the bathroom/leave/etc."

File

Where you go from here is up to you and depends on several factors including your confidence level, the discriminating party, and your state. Different states have different enforcement provisions (or lack thereof) for their laws. In California, you can file a civil complaint[22] of discrimination under the Unruh Civil Rights Act. "I will leave now, but I will be filing a legal complaint of discrimination under the Unruh Civil Rights Act." Best for Babes has a Nursing in Public Discrimination hotline you can call where you can be put in touch with support and resources in your area.[34] Document everything, and you can consult an attorney if you feel it is necessary. If you are unsure if discrimination has actually taken place, ask yourself this: would a bottle-feeding parent have been restricted in the same manner? If you are being treated differently (unjustly) due to your breastfeeding status, which is a biological function of being a woman, that is sex discrimination.

Stand Up

I so encourage you to stand up for yourself and your baby. The simple act of calmly asserting your legal right to breastfeed in public can pave the way for all of the breastfeeding mothers and babies to follow behind you. You don't have to "win." You just have to breastfeed your baby at the front of the bus. Regardless of the outcome, that is the victory—just walking the path and using your voice simply to state that your baby has a right to eat if/when the need arises.

Support

For those of you reading this chapter who are not presently lactating, your role in normalizing breastfeeding and supporting breastfeeding mothers is just as vital for breastfeeding success. You are the partner in this dance. You can improve breastfeeding rates, which have substantial benefits for Baby (example: higher IQ for each month of breastfeeding[23]), Mother (example: reduced risk of breast cancer[24]), and society at large (example: reduced costs to tax payers—$13 billion if 90% of babies were breastfed[25]) by accepting breastfeeding without condition. There is no threshold of cover, location, or age at which breastfeeding in public is inappropriate. It is *always* appropriate. Communicating this through your words and actions will set us all up for success. Simply smile at a breastfeeding mama, treat her like a normal human being (and not a leper), offer to open a door for her or pick up something she drops, offer her a water, and stand with her in defense of her rights if/when necessary.

Partners/husbands/co-parents in particular have a powerful role in the ease or stress and difficulty of breastfeeding in public. Having a copilot at your side to assist and support you in every way can literally be the deal breaker in achieving your breastfeeding goals or not. Sometimes husbands can be led astray by feelings that are based on a false sense of ownership over their wives' bodies. She chooses to share her body with you. She chooses to share her body with her baby. She is the sole owner of her body and she alone can decide what is appropriate and comfortable for her. And remember, if every feeding outside of the house is wrought with tension, your baby is receiving those stress hormones too. It is important for your partner to be just as educated as you about breastfeeding. Can a plane fly with one pilot? Sure, but this is a long flight. Having your mate there to bring you a glass of water, suggest a course change, or settle a disgruntled passenger means everything. Breastfeeding can strengthen a marriage or weaken it. It's up to you, partner: Who do you choose to be for your baby and wife? She will remember this dynamic for the rest of her life.

Altogether

Anxiety around breastfeeding in public can lead to isolation, breed depression, and reduce the chances of breastfeeding success. So shed it. Ain't no shame in your game! Breastfeeding in public is just breastfeeding; it is simply an extension of your existing breastfeeding relationship. It is you living your life with your baby—nothing more, nothing less. What do you choose to make of that life?

4

FULL-TERM BREASTFEEDING

So you have committed to breastfeeding. You are embracing the physical and psychological benefits for your baby that honor their emotional and nutritional needs. But for how long? As with so many aspects of motherhood, I encourage you to look to your child and trust in their wisdom.

Natural Progression

We are genetically programed to thrive on Mama's milk. And this truth extends beyond the 12-months mark. Most mothers who breastfeed for a period of years don't set out specifically to do so. They celebrate their child's first birthday, and the next morning, when that beautifully innocent and perfect face lovingly nuzzles into their chest with trust and peace and joy, it just doesn't make sense that it was good yesterday but now, somehow, bad today. A little research later, they are able to continue their breastfeeding relationship confident that it *does* continue to be mutually beneficial until the child naturally weans.

Evolution

"Full-term" breastfeeding is referred to as such because it means to breastfeed your child for the full duration, as is natural and healthy for our species. While the age at which any individual child initiates weaning from the breast can vary widely, the species average is about 4. Think about it; children lose their baby teeth, or "milk teeth," at around the age of 6 (age at which they get their first adult molar, which is the point at which primates naturally wean),[57] and a child's immune system is not fully formed until around the age of 6 (the mother's immune system provides the needed antibodies prior to this milestone).[58] Did I just lose you? Don't jump the train! Full-term breastfeeding is *not* about any sensationalized image that may have just come into your head. It is simply about continuing to breastfeed for as long as feels right for you and your child (not prematurely severing the breastfeeding relationship based on an arbitrary date or milestone), accepting that the health benefits to doing so continue beyond infancy.

Official Recommendations

The World Health Organization (WHO) officially recommends, "Exclusive breastfeeding . . . up to 6 months of age, with continued breastfeeding along with appropriate complementary foods up to two years of age or beyond."[2] The American Academy of Pediatrics (AAP) recommends, " . . . exclusive breastfeeding for about the first six months of a baby's life, followed by breastfeeding in combination with the introduction of complementary foods until at least 12 months of age, and continuation of breastfeeding for as long as mutually desired by mother and baby."[3]

Physical Benefits

Both of these policy statements on duration of breastfeeding use language that acknowledges the continued benefit of breastfeeding beyond infancy, for as long as is mutually desired. "Breastmilk is, after all, milk. Even after six months, it still contains protein, fat, and other nutritionally important and appropriate elements which babies and children need. Breastmilk still contains immunologic factors that help protect the child even if he is 2 or older. In fact, some immune factors in breastmilk that protect the baby against infection are present in greater amounts in the second year of life than in the first. This is, of course as it should be, since children older than a year are generally exposed to more infections than young babies. Breastmilk still contains special growth factors that help the immune system to mature, and which help the brain, gut, and other organs to develop and mature."[4]

Psychological Benefits

The psychological benefit of the continuation of the breastfeeding relationship until the child steps away is priceless. Breastfeeding is so much more to a child than a source of perfect nutrition. Feeding at the breast fills their entire being. A 2-year-old who awoke from a bad dream is instantly comforted back into security with some nighttime nursing. Breastfeeding a child doesn't take away from—it adds to. It does not inhibit independence. *Independence is not taught—it blooms.* Allowing your child to fill up their belly and their love cup until satiated is a gift that can yield returns in the form of a content, secure, heart-full child. Having the healing comfort of breastmilk for your fevered child can make all the difference for you both. It can add to what you have to offer your child without becoming a burden.

Benefits for Mother

Full-term breastfeeding also has direct physical benefits for you. One of my favorite benefits is the delayed return of Aunt Flow. My period did not return after my third child until 26 months postpartum (Score!). This also means that breastfeeding acts as a form of birth control. If you are ecologically breastfeeding (breastfeeding in the fashion described in this book, utilizing tenets such as breastfeeding on cue, night nursing, no supplemental sucking, etc.), then your body recognizes that your baby's level of need is still too high to allow for a sibling. Brilliant, right?! Of course, I don't want to be responsible for any unplanned pregnancies, so I do have to caution you that you can ovulate before you see the return of your period. The literature tells us that for the first 6 months postpartum, if you are ecologically breastfeeding, " . . . the chances of pregnancy are less than two percent, making it a more reliable birth-spacing method than a condom or a diaphragm."[60] (Though, admittedly, I wouldn't let my husband even wink in my general direction without another form of birth control!)

But my favorite physical benefit for Mom has to be the significantly reduced risk for breast cancer. A Yale study found that breastfeeding for 2 years reduced the risk by 50%[62] while a meta analysis found that the risk was reduced for each month of breastfeeding.[61] So for every month I give my growing little one this powerful gift for his health, I am also giving to myself.

Fertility

If you have embraced full-term breastfeeding and wish to add to your brood, you can coax the return of your menstrual cycle by dialing back the nursing sessions. Some women wonder if breastfeeding while pregnant is possible or advisable. You can stay calm and breastfeed on confidently with the knowledge that there is no evidence that suggests that it is unsafe or unhealthy to breastfeed while pregnant.[59] That said, it is always a good idea to discuss any concerns you might have with your health care provider, particularly if you have a history of preterm labor (as there is a relationship between nipple stimulation and contractions). Many women report an agitated feeling while breastfeeding during pregnancy that is due to the fact that your nipples are extra sensitive during the first trimester. In fact, many a mother has realized she is pregnant due to this phenomenon. By mid-pregnancy, the majority of women experience a significant drop in milk supply. For some little ones, this change leads to weaning. For those little ones who continue, you will likely be stepping into tandem nursing.

Tandem Nursing

Tandem nursing is the term for breastfeeding two children at the same time. One major benefit for Mom when adding a second nursling is that you don't have any of the uncomfortable challenges associated with the early weeks of breastfeeding such as engorgement or sore nipples, since your breasts are already in full lactation mode. And since your supply will adjust to and meet the demand, there should be ample milky goodness for all your loves. Just be sure that your newborn gets first dibs, as your older child benefits from the nutritional complement of solid foods. I have found that this shared, special mommy real estate really enhances the bond between siblings.

Weaning

If you reach the point when you are ready for a child to wean before your child begins to taper interest, honor those feelings within yourself. Breastfeeding is a *relationship,* and any discomfort or resentment that could stem from ignoring those feelings within you will no longer be enhancing your relationship. Do a little soul-searching and uncover the root of your discomfort. If it is coming from somewhere outside you and your breastfeeding child, try not to let it taint something that is pure and good for all the parties that matter in this equation. If, after getting in touch with those feelings, you realize that you are ready to transition away from the breastfeeding relationship, consider using a gentle transition:

- Don't offer, don't refuse. Don't present your child with the breast, but at the same time, allow for breastfeeding when requested.
- Avoid situations associated with breastfeeding. If you have spent the last three years rocking in the bedroom rocking chair with a quilt for nursing, don't spend hours each day and night in that rocking chair, cuddled with that quilt, annoyed that your child wants to breastfeed.
- Shift your bedtime routine and build it around other attachment centered activities like cuddling in bed while reading stories, rubbing their back, etc.
- Keep busy. While at home, my toddler would spend most of his time cuddled up and attached to me. However, when out and about, adventuring in the world, he would easily go all day without even thinking about breastfeeding.
- Expect that your child may cling to a favorite feeding (like the last nursing session of the evening or the first one after waking) and that their appetite for breastfeeding will increase during times of pain, illness, or distress.

My first nursling weaned at a year. I continued to offer and was always intent on allowing his needs to guide our breastfeeding relationship. But right around his first birthday, he was done. Looking back, I can see many factors that contributed to his weaning such as his voracious appetite for food, his desire for stimulating activities, my absence while in grad school, my placement of a blanket over his head anytime he wanted to breastfeed in public (which was harder and more stressful for us both), not co-sleeping around this time period, and night weaning. I can look back and wonder how much of a role these factors and others played in his weaning process, but at the end of the day, I have to tell myself that I did the best I could with the information I had at the time and be proud of that gift of a year of on-cue breastfeeding (exclusively for the first 6 months) I lovingly gave my first baby.

I don't regret one single second of the over three and a half years I spent breastfeeding my sweet Bay. Those days and nights cuddled together, him smiling around his latch, those big brown eyes gazing up at me, beaming pure happiness, were perfect. Perfect for him. Perfect for me. Perfect for us. The world could have crumbled around us and all he would have needed to insulate himself from any discontent would be to connect in this special way, his face resting on my chest. He really didn't even eat much food before he was about 18 months old. As he matured, breastfeeding became his efficient means of filling up his love cup so he could bravely launch out into the world in independent exploration. Ten minutes of breastfeeding could fuel him for hours and hours of risk taking and new friend making. He breastfed while I was pregnant with his brother. We tandem nursed for a brief time in perfect harmony. I did feel a little alone sometimes, but I sought support from other full-term breastfeeders and was steadfast in my trust in his journey. We were both very happy and healthy, and that is what mattered. Eventually, he was only breastfeeding at bedtime and morning time. Then he was just cuddling his "night-night milks" at nighttime. Until one day we both realized he had weaned. The Hebrew word for wean translates as "to ripen." My Mana, Bay, was ripe. I will breastfeed my West full term. I will honor whatever that means for him. But I look forward to years of adventuring in the world with a nursling in the pouch. I will enjoy and appreciate every moment of connection that fulfills him so completely in this special way. And the day he walks over the threshold of our home as a man, I will smile, confident that I nourished his body and soul to the fullest.

Support

Only 16.4% of American mothers exclusively breastfeed for at least 6 months[65] despite all the overwhelming evidence of the significant benefits to both Baby and Mother and the official recommendations of every official department or organization that makes recommendations on such matters. The normalization of breastfeeding is going a long way in shifting the tide by establishing an informal shared knowledge base and network of social support. But to truly see marked gains in women being able to meet their breastfeeding goals, significant changes need to be made on a larger scale. First, the US needs to comply with the WHO code prohibiting formula marketing, sampling, and physician bribery. Second, the US must have paid maternity leave (which is present in virtually all industrialized nations) so that women have enough time to anchor their breastfeeding relationship before returning to work. Third, health care providers need to be educated in breastfeeding. Presently, doctors receive virtually no education or training in the physiology of breastfeeding and treatment of any potential problems. Fourth, every state needs laws protecting a woman's right to nurse in public, along with accompanying enforcement provisions, which would provide consequences for breastfeeding discrimination.[67]

Altogether

Breastfeeding for four weeks or four years is a gift. My hope for the world is that breastfeeding will be considered the normal, expected way to feed a child and our culture will reflect support of that ideal. My hope for you is that you are freed from any sense of taboo or weight of arbitrary deadlines to focus on what is there between you and your child; what continues to flourish when you breastfeed your child until they are body and heart full.

5

MISCONCEPTIONS ABOUT THE ALMIGHTY BOOB

Most women don't produce enough milk.

The vast majority of women *do* produce just the right amount of milk for their babies, no supplementing required. However, it is a common fear among moms that their babies are not getting enough milk. Out of a desire to ensure the very best for our babies, we try to control and manage even natural processes that function best when not micromanaged. If your pediatrician is concerned about your baby's slow weight gain, ensure that your doctor is referencing the World Heath Organization's (WHO) Breastfeeding Infant's Growth Chart (not the Centers for Disease Control and Prevention's (CDC), which is based on formula-fed infants).[5, 30] You can spend more time skin-to-skin, drink plenty of water, and offer the breast frequently to encourage feeding. You can also meet with a quality lactation consultant at a breastfeeding support group or in a private consultation. There are many avenues you can pursue for stimulating more production. But the best thing you can do is *relax* and trust in your body.

If you can't produce enough or any breastmilk for your baby, formula is your only option.

There are some amazing mamas out there who donate their excess breastmilk. You can go through a milk bank or join a direct milk sharing organization.[9] A milk bank processes and screens their milk. This process kills some of the living components of the breastmilk, and milk banks tend to be pricey. With direct milk sharing, you are using milk that that mother is feeding her own baby (can't get much better of an endorsement than that) and you can flash boil the received donated milk in a process that would kill even HIV.

You know the milk you buy from the grocery store is a cow's breastmilk, right? It comes from a dirty, stinky farm animal and is tailor-made for baby cows. My breastmilk is tailor-made for baby *humans*. Were I overproducing with a stockpile in the freezer, I would happily donate that extra breastmilk to an under- or non-producing mom or dad. We transplant organs, we transfuse blood, we share milk.

Cross nursing can also be a good resource among close friends. Need to leave your baby with a mama friend for a few hours? She could nurse your baby alongside her own and vice versa.

Pumping will show me how much milk I am producing.

Pumping is not an accurate indicator of how much breastmilk your baby is receiving. Pumps are not babies and your brilliant breasts know the difference. Instead, weigh your baby before a feeding, then after (you can stand on your scale and subtract your baby's weight from your own) and you will get a more accurate picture.

Larger breasts produce more milk.

More breast tissue (fat) does not equal a greater volume of milk glands.[6] A woman with larger breasts can have a low supply and a woman with smaller breasts can have an over supply. If you do have a smaller milk storage capacity, your baby will likely just feed more frequently. My very humble breasts "rocked the Casbah,"[10] exclusively breastfeeding three babies on cue for a combined ten years and counting. Have I mentioned that my first and third babies were 20 pounds at 3 months old?

Breastfeeding is more work.

Breastfeeding is the lazy mom's best friend! My formula-feeding friend might have to wake up at 2 a.m., walk to the kitchen, take out a bottle and sterilized artificial nipple, get the formula, mix formula with water, heat it, feed the baby, put the baby back to sleep, go back to the kitchen and wash the dishes. I roll over and he opens his mouth. Done! I can make milk and feed my baby while I am sleeping. No bottles to wash, no artificial nipples to sterilize, no formula to buy (a hefty expense). I open my shirt and snap down my bra—lazy mom's dream come true.

It is easier to bottle-feed in public.

Think about all the gear required to bottle-feed out in the world that you must carry with you at all times: bottle, artificial nipple, cap, formula container with formula, purified water, and a means to heat that formula once mixed. Again, the breastfeeding process consists simply of opening the shirt and bra you are already wearing. Read the Nursing in Public chapter for more on this topic.

You can't leave the house if you breastfeed.

This is terrible advice. I love my house, but no matter how lovely, I still wouldn't want to be imprisoned in it. You *absolutely* can and should leave the house. Breastfeeding is extremely society friendly. It keeps babies content and happy while being extremely convenient. Lunch is always ready at Mama's Milk Diner. Again, read the Nursing in Public chapter for more on this topic.

You can never leave a breastfeeding child.

While the supply and demand system of breastfeeding does function optimally when mother and baby are together, you are free to separate as much or as little as with a formula-fed baby. Pump some milk into a bottle with a simple hand pump. You have just as much or as little freedom of independence as any new mother.

A breastfeeding mother can never consume alcohol.

The greatest risk posed to an infant with an intoxicated mother is being dropped or suffocated due to Mom's loss of motor coordination. Alcohol content in breastmilk mirrors alcohol in blood. This means that as your liver processes the alcohol, your milk gets sober too.[71]

I have to quit breastfeeding to take a medication (my doctor told me so).

I strongly encourage you to check every medication you are prescribed in Dr. Hale's book *Medications and Mother's Milk*, with the Infant Risk Hotline, or on the LactMed app.[73, 74, 75] It's a simple matter of looking up the medication prescribed and checking the safety rating. If only I could get these resources into the hands of every physician so they would stop telling nursing women to prematurely and unnecessarily wean to take medication that is actually safe while breastfeeding.

Breastmilk and formula are comparable.

Not even close. Breastmilk is full of antibodies, hormones, anti-viruses, anti-allergies, anti-parasites, growth factors, and enzymes completely absent from formula. Formula-fed babies are at greater risk for ear infections, respiratory infections, meningitis, diarrhea/constipation, pneumonia, Sudden Infant Death Syndrome (SIDS), and of developing obesity, diabetes, asthma, allergies, cancer and a lower IQ.[11, 12] And newly researched benefits of breastmilk are discovered every day. Formula companies try to duplicate the ingredients but they just can't even come close. Looking at a complete list of known ingredients, the formula column pales in comparison.[13]

It's a good idea to keep that free formula sample—just in case.

"Research shows that the main factor in continued breastfeeding is whether a woman exclusively breastfeeds at the hospital or not . . . 'Formula samples received from a medical facility signals to the mom that formula feeding is medically endorsed' . . . 16.4% of American mothers exclusively breastfeed for at least six months."[65]

Throw it away. The numbers are clear: If a family is given and accepts a free formula sample, Mom is less likely to successfully breastfeed. You will likely turn to the formula instead of breastfeeding support during any challenges along your breastfeeding journey.

If you choose to breastfeed, you need to supplement with formula and vitamins for your baby to receive all the proper nutrients.

Unless your baby has been identified as having a specific problem for which a specific supplement has been recommended, breastmilk is all your baby needs. If a specific recommendation is made, I urge you to thoroughly research outcomes and make informed choices for your baby.[8]

Breastfeeding comes completely naturally.

Some aspects of breastfeeding knowledge fall into the innate column. For example, newborn infants will use their stepping reflex to make their way up Mommy's body toward the bull's-eye created by the enlarged areola and darkened nipple and start sucking as the nipple triggers their rooting reflex. Some aspects of breastfeeding are learned, like positioning and optimal latch. I once read a fitting metaphor comparing breastfeeding to riding a bike. You live your life having never seen anyone ride a bike (or while they rode they were covered from the neck down by a blanket) or receiving any instruction, and on the day your baby is born you are given a bike and pushed down a hill. If we do not grow up with breastfeeding role models around us (read the Nursing in Public chapter for more about the importance of breastfeeding in public for normalizing breastfeeding) nor receive any formal education on the process, the chances for successfully reaching our breastfeeding goals are low. And that's not even taking into account the forces of an unsupportive society and targeted formula marketing. Breastfeeding *is* natural and once you get your riding legs, it *feels* natural.

You are a failure as a mother if you cannot or do not

breastfeed.

Babies are supposed to be born the way Mother Nature intended: through the birth canal. Sometimes physical conditions arise in which a vaginal birth is physically not a safe option. Thankfully, under those circumstances, we have surgical technology and skilled doctors available to us to perform c-sections. The same can be said of breastfeeding. Babies are supposed to be fed at the breast with breastmilk as Mother Nature designed. Many mothers who formula-feed do so as a result of a lack of support and dedication. Sometimes, on rare occasions, conditions arise in which breastfeeding is not an option, even with all the supportive forces in the world. Thankfully, under those circumstances, we have donated breastmilk and/or formula to feed our babies. Gratitude and pride is what I feel toward women who are able to take what they have been dealt and utilize the resources at their disposal to make the best choices for their babies with peace and confidence. To be clear: you are not a failure.

If your milk doesn't come in right away, you won't produce any.

I had a friend who, after the premature birth of her baby, was told by the hospital's lactation consultant that if days after her traumatic surgical birth she wasn't producing milk, it would never come in, and she needed to let it go. Insert my dropped jaw here. Thankfully, she was educated and experienced enough with breastfeeding (and had me yell texting with her husband) to stick with it, and over a year later, she is still enjoying a perfect breastfeeding relationship with her baby.

Your body makes your baby's first milk, colostrum, while you are pregnant. It usually takes three to four days for your milk to surge in volume, but it can take up to a week.[7] All of those attachment-promoting behaviors involved in kangaroo care (keeping Baby skin-to-skin on your chest) can help to bring your milk strongly and quickly.

Baby has acid reflux if they cry, spit up, and don't sleep through the night.

Your baby is a human infant if they cry, spit up, and don't sleep through the night. This is an issue that has begun to weigh heavily on my mind, as there is suddenly a huge spike in the number of babies in my Sage Baby classes that are on acid reflux medications. Babies are being diagnosed with acid reflux and put on serious medication (an off-label use) that has significant side effects (for example, food allergies) when parents present their infants to the pediatrician with symptoms of crying, spitting up, and not sleeping enough (all of which are *normal* symptoms of infancy, in varying degrees), looking for their baby to be fixed. Studies are showing that while the PPI's (proton-pump inhibitors) are reducing (healthy) acid content in the stomach, they are having *no* effect on the presenting symptoms. As one doctor puts it, "We are medicalizing normality." This is not to say that there are no legitimate cases of GERD (Gastroesophageal Reflux Disease), but it is vastly over diagnosed and over medicated.[35]

There is nothing you can do to help a baby with a troubled tummy.

Learn how to properly massage that belly in an infant massage class like Sage Baby![44] I like to tell parents that any compassionate touch is good touch, and if Baby is happy and you are happy, then you are doing it right. The only exception to this is over the belly because you have to move in the directions of digestion to really move things through and pick up the efficiency of the digestive system. Once you learn the proper strokes (think clockwise and down), you can move through a week of constipation in one fell swoop, and you can work out a gassy tummy with nothing more than your loving touch. It's an incredible and powerful thing.

The other suggestion I have for a little troubled tummy is to wear your baby chest-to-chest. Babywearing in this position keeps your baby upright (keeps things moving down), applies comforting pressure to your baby's abdomen, and provides rhythmic movement (works out obstructions), all while in your loving embrace and providing you the convenience of mobility and free hands.

Could your baby have sensitivity to a food in your diet? "If a breastfed baby is sensitive to a particular food, then he may be fussy after feedings, cry inconsolably for long periods, or sleep little and wake suddenly with obvious discomfort. There may be a family history of allergies. Other signs of a food allergy may include: rash, hives, eczema, sore bottom, dry skin; wheezing or asthma; congestion or cold-like symptoms; red, itchy eyes; ear infections; irritability, fussiness, colic; intestinal upsets, vomiting, constipation and/or diarrhea, or green stools with mucus or blood."[47] Food allergies in a breastfed baby are not a death sentence for breastfeeding. If you suspect a particular food as the culprit, for example dairy, which is the most common food allergy for the breastfed baby, completely eliminate it from your diet for two weeks. If your baby's symptoms go away, then stay dairy free. If they persist, eliminate the next suspect for two weeks.

You must work to ensure a proper foremilk/hindmilk balance.

Foremilk is the milk that is sitting at the forefront of your breasts and is consumed by your baby at the start of breastfeeding, which is typically higher in sugar and water content. Hindmilk is the milk further back in the breast, which is typically higher in fat and protein content (looks creamier). Nurslings thrive on a mixture of both and there is absolutely nothing that the typical mother needs to do to ensure an ideal mix. No, you do not need to do anything to ensure a proper foremilk/hindmilk balance.

If you are engorged with an over supply and your baby has explosive, foamy green poop along with gas, bloating, abdominal distention, or reflux, then you could have a foremilk/hindmilk imbalance. For most, this means your baby is getting mostly foremilk and is full before getting to that hindmilk. Thankfully, the treatment is harmless and easily tried to see if it alleviates your baby's gastrointestinal discomfort. The first strategy is to breastfeed your baby on the same side for every feeding in one day and pump the other side. Then switch the next day (block nursing). The second strategy is to simply pump n' dump for a few minutes before breastfeeding your baby. Try this for several days and see if it makes a difference. If it does, then continue until you balance out (and you will eventually achieve balance). If not, then it is probably not a case of a foremilk/hindmilk imbalance and you may want to consider eliminations from your diet to check for potential allergies.[43]

An improper latch means you must quit breastfeeding.

If you are struggling with an ineffective and painful latch, I urge you to seek the help of a lactation consultant (IBCLC (International Board Certified Lactation Consultant)). One note on lactation consultants: some are amazing and some are not. If the first does not provide the support you need, get some recommendations and try another. It is worth it. You can also find significant help at a breastfeeding support group. Many are even no or low cost.

One common cause of latch problems is a tongue or lip tie (which can be diagnosed by an IBCLC). A tongue tie exists when the frenum is attached too far toward the tip of the tongue. This causes limited mobility of the tongue, which is a main player in the act of breastfeeding (as the latch is actually created with the tongue, not the lower lip). A lip tie exists when tissue connects the upper lip far down the gum line where the upper teeth will eventually emerge. A lip tie prevents the upper lip from opening wide enough to maintain a good latch. In both cases, a pediatric dentist or ear, nose, and throat doctor can release the tie by cutting or with a laser.[46]

Sleep training does not affect breastfeeding.

Night waking from hunger is not a behavioral issue; it is a physical need. You cannot teach your baby to have a bigger stomach. At one month of age, your baby's stomach is still only the size of an egg.[36] This means that they cannot store enough milk to last all through the night. So if you're sleep training, you are forcing your baby to sit in a torturous state of hunger for a prolonged period of time, which can have significant consequences for overall health from lack of nutrition, such as Failure to Thrive (FTT). You are also damaging the foundation of trust (communication yields response) that is essential to the cooperative breastfeeding relationship (demand yields supply). In addition to the negative effects on Baby's end of the breastfeeding relationship, there is a significant pitfall for you as the milk producer: Breastmilk production is highest at night, so skipping the night nursing will significantly reduce your overall milk production.

You cannot breastfeed if you have had breast augmentation.

Yes, you can breastfeed if you have had breast implants or a breast reduction. A lot of the specifics depend on your particular situation, so do some homework to see how you can overcome your specific challenges.[45]

Dad won't be able to bond with the baby if you breastfeed.

There are so many ways in which Daddy can bond with his baby: kangaroo care, babywearing, infant massage, singing and dancing with Baby, responding sensitively and consistently to Baby's cues, bathing with Baby, etc. To say that a daddy cannot have a strong bond with his breastfed baby is completely false. My husband has never fed our little West and enjoys an extremely close bond with him—as his daddy. He is not Mommy; he is Daddy. He does not make milk or have boob pillows on his chest. Daddy likes to run and jump, his voice has the low hum of a deep drum, and we love to stick our tongues out at each other.

Lactating is a biological function of a woman's breasts. This is not a sexist denial of men. Breastfeeding is one of a myriad of ways to bond with a baby, to which Daddy has full access.

Breastfeeding is easy.
Breastfeeding is hard.

You should not underestimate the dedication and support required to successfully breastfeed, nor should you be intimidated by a perceived high level of difficulty. Educate yourself and have some supportive resources in place. Pair this with trust in yourself—a belief that you can and will breastfeed just fine—and a commitment to follow through—you will breastfeed your baby despite any challenges that do arise.

My first baby breastfed like a champ from minutes

after birth. I was challenged by painful, engorged breasts and cracked, bleeding nipples for the first couple weeks (along with after pains that accompanied letdown). Those free formula samples looked enticing. I threw them away, researched some remedies, talked with my sister (who breastfed her four kids), and after a couple weeks, my body had adjusted. I have since enjoyed a decade of effortless and rewarding breastfeeding.

If you get mastitis, you have to stop breastfeeding and take antibiotics.

"Mastitis is an infection of the breast tissue that results in breast pain, swelling, warmth and redness of the breast. If you have mastitis, you might also experience fever and chills."[42] The absolute best thing you can do for mastitis is breastfeed, breastfeed, breastfeed! Think of a river flowing out through your ducts, clearing your breast of the mastitis. Also, stay completely topless to avoid any binding and increase ventilation around the breast and nipple. Hot showers and massaging the breast are also helpful. Husbands are usually pretty big fans of this treatment course: "My wife needs to stay topless, take steamy showers, and have someone massage her breasts? I volunteer." Eating garlic, taking vitamin C, and drinking *tons* of water while getting lots of rest with baby is the best medicine. If some time passes and your state is not improving, then you can seek a prescription for antibiotics from a doctor.

If you wish to become pregnant, you must cease breastfeeding.

It is true that one of the fantastic benefits of full-term breastfeeding is that it can act as a natural birth control. But if fertility is your goal, you can encourage ovulation by breastfeeding *less*—far from weaning completely. You can also breastfeed while pregnant, and even tandem nurse. You can read more about the relationship between breastfeeding and pregnancy in the Full-Term Breastfeeding chapter.

You should not be a human pacifier.

Let's really think about this for a minute. The pacifier being referred to is an imitation nipple. So you're advising not to be a real, fake . . . you? How is the absurdity of this lost on some people? The spirit of this warning is that you should only allow your baby to breastfeed for strictly physical, nutritionally based reasons. You cannot isolate the moment-to-moment motivations for breastfeeding! Babies breastfeed for all of the benefits in a completely interconnected way. Deny your baby the breast because you perceive they are receiving primarily comfort and you deny your baby milk and a significant portion of the overall benefits to breastfeeding. It's that simple.

Night nursing causes cavities.

Cavities, or dental caries, are caused by a bacterium called strep mutans, which produces acid that causes decay. Breastmilk contains lactoferrin, which actually kills strep mutans. Based on all available research, Pediatric Dentistry stated that, "It is concluded that human breast milk is not cariogenic,"[63] and the American Dental Association proclaimed that there is " . . . no association between breastfeeding and early childhood caries."[64]

Bottle rot is a condition of childhood tooth decay where a formula- (or cow's milk-) fed child sleeps with a bottle in their mouth. The formula (or cow's milk) pours from the artificial nipple and pools in the mouth, resting on the teeth all night long. The mechanics of breastfeeding differ in that a child must be actively sucking to pull the breastmilk into his mouth (no milk passively dripping all night long) and the nipple is placed well behind the teeth. The strep mutans bacterium can be introduced into the mouth through artificial nipples and bottles, and the dietary components of the formula, cow's milk, or other foods in the child's diet (sugar) all contribute to the formation of cavities while simultaneously lacking the lactoferrin, milk protein (which protects enamel), and antibacterial components of breastmilk.

Breastfeeding is psychosexually damaging, especially beyond a certain age.

As was discussed in the Nursing in Public chapter, breastfeeding for a few years is the norm for a homo sapien. Both mother and child are evolutionarily designed to thrive under that condition and within that breastfeeding relationship. There is no research that exists showing any negative effect from breastfeeding beyond any milestone or age. Laws and official recommendations reflect this (supporting a woman's right to breastfeed her child for as long as is mutually desired by both parties). Uninformed opinions, judgments, and gossip may not, but thankfully, I don't base my parenting decisions on those things.

Breastfeeding past a year is more for the mother than the baby.
Once you can ask for it, you're too old for it.
Once they have teeth, Baby needs to be cut off.

Breastfeeding is not fantastically healthy the day your baby is 11 months and 29 days old and then disgustingly unhealthy the day your baby is 12 months old. Verbal ability and presence of teeth are irrelevant. Some kids don't talk until they are a couple years old. Some babies are born with teeth. Ignore the little quips and do what feels right for your child knowing that science supports the luck of a baby who enjoys an extended breastfeeding relationship. Read the Full-Term Breastfeeding chapter for more on this topic.

6

BOTTLE-FEEDING WITH BREASTFEEDING STYLE

Although the benefits of breastfeeding are immense, you may find yourself in the position of bottle-feeding expressed breastmilk or formula. Parents find themselves in this position for a variety of reasons. In rare circumstances, it is in the best interest of your baby to be bottle-fed. One such example might be a mother who is on medication that is not safe for Baby but that she requires in order to care for Baby. Another example might be a mother who has chosen to return to work but wishes to continue giving her baby the gift of pumped breastmilk.

Many mothers who find themselves with a bottle in their hands have merely fallen into the booby traps. Negative factors such as a lack of role modeling, public and/or family support, and educational/technical support, along with positive factors (positive meaning a presence of as opposed to a lack of) like free formula samples, media portrayals of infant feeding, and the challenges of the first weeks of breastfeeding, all make a trail leading to formula-feeding. I urge you to accept breastfeeding as the way your baby was made to eat and what your breasts were made for, and breastmilk as the food millions of years of evolution tailor-made to give your baby every advantage. I encourage you to exhaust every avenue of support before formula-feeding because the lifelong benefit to your baby (and you) is worth overcoming a lot, especially since the vast majority of breastfeeding challenges can be overcome. If you are among the very small minority of women who decide that breastfeeding is not possible for you or not in the best interest of your baby, you can capture some of the benefits of the breastfeeding relationship by tapping into some of the breastfeeding style and strategies.

On Cue

One aspect of infant feeding that is common to the breastfeeding relationship is feeding on cue. Baby gives a cue that they would like to feed and Mom puts Baby at the breast. When parents are bottle-feeding they tend to fall into scheduling. There are many things that contribute to this tendency such as the inconvenience of the supplies and preparation required for bottle-feeding, the involvement of numerous feeders (other than mom), the disconnect that can manifest between a parent and a baby who are not directly physically responding to each other, etc. Feeding on cue tunes parents in to the cues of their baby and they then read and respond to those cues through feeding. This begins with feeding your baby and extends to the length of each feeding. Most breastfeeding mothers offer milk when Baby displays a cue that they want to breastfeed and withdraw the breast as soon as they display a cue that they are done. If you have just done all the work (and shouldered the financial expense) of preparing a bottle, you will tend not to want to stop before the bottle is emptied. If you can forget about the measurement lines on the bottle and ignore the clock, feeding your baby on cue, you can tap into one of the bond-strengthening benefits of breastfeeding while bottle-feeding.

Positioning

When a mother and baby breastfeed, the baby's face and mother's face are roughly 6–12 inches apart—the exact distance to which a newborn can see. Nature designed your baby's view at the breast to maximize bonding and learning. While a breastfed baby is breastfeeding, Mom's face is center stage, and with those big, innocent eyes gazing at them, they tend to be happy to take full advantage of the captive audience. As the two stare into each other's eyes for hours throughout the day and night, magic things happen. For example: Mom talks to her baby in that special way that moms do (Motherese), expressively speaking to Baby in a way that captures their attention and teaches them the foundation of language. This benefit of the breastfeeding relationship can be tapped into while bottle-feeding if you simply lay the bottle right on your breast or hold it against your chest at a similar angle. Holding the bottle in the same position as the breast every time you feed your baby sets you and your baby up for all the same face-to-face interaction that takes place during breastfeeding. It also allows your baby to utilize one of their natural regulators of overstimulation. Babies frequently breastfeed when in an overstimulating situation because it turns them away from the world, focusing them right in on their emotional anchor: you.

Breaks

Additionally, being able to turn away from the tap helps babies learn to self-regulate their food intake. When a breastfeeding baby needs a breather, they simply turn away and take a break. This break can allow them to catch their breath and check in with their hunger. Do they want more? Are they full? So keep the bottle stationary and *don't follow your baby with the bottle when they turn their head*. Eating while being stimulated results in overeating, just as research tells us that adults eating in front of the television overeat. If your baby is facing out while eating they are focused on all of the stimulation around them and not on the job at hand, which is to listen to the cues of their body and eat to satisfaction. Also, if your baby becomes accustomed to eating while interacting with the rest of the world (facing out), they may resist nursing, which requires tuning out the busy world and focusing inward. Along these lines, be sure to *never* bottle prop. Bottle propping is the act of propping the bottle in your baby's mouth so they are being fed without you. Babies have died from bottle propping and it can lead to ear infections and bottle caries. When a bottle is propped, there is no one reading all of your baby's cues as they eat, which is not safe.[38]

Alternate

Another beneficial aspect of natural breastfeeding positioning is that we alternate sides equally. This results in babies' eyes and necks being exercised in both directions (as they orient toward the direction of the mother). While bottle-feeding, caregivers frequently hold babies in their left arms to feed with their right (dominant) hand. Falling into this single-sided arrangement can also lead to a side preference while breastfeeding, which can cause problems for Mom when breastfeeding straight from the tap.

Contact

One powerful source of bonding between a mother and baby is all of the skin-to-skin contact that is a part of breastfeeding. It is a common occurrence between a breastfeeding mom and baby to spend all day shirtless and connected. If you are bottle-feeding, it may seem odd to spend time shirtless, but skin-to-skin contact is powerfully nurturing to your baby's body. So as often as you can, be home, shirtless, and glued to each other in oxytocin bliss.

Closeness

Proximity is a cornerstone of every breastfeeding relationship. In order to produce milk, you have to sense the demand, and in order to respond to your baby's cues of hunger, you have to be in close proximity to your baby at almost all times. Since bottle-feeding moms have the "freedom" of not being physically tethered to their babies, they tend to allow more time and space between themselves and their babies. Your baby benefits greatly from your presence. It's as simple as that. Realize that your physical presence is just as essential for your baby when bottle-feeding as when breastfeeding and you give your baby another benefit commonly enjoyed by breastfeeding babies.

Pumping

If you are returning to work or doing something else that is requiring a significant amount of time away from your baby, you may find your supply suffering as you pump to provide milk for your little one. So here are some tips to keep in mind for successfully pumping:

> Allergy meds do decrease supply. If your supply is ample and you increase your water intake, you may be fine taking the allergy meds while lactating. However, if you are trying to increase

your supply, know that allergy meds dry up body fluids; that's partly how they do their job.

Prolactin (milk-producing hormone) levels are highest during the night, so if you are trying to pump and struggling to get enough for your baby during the day, add a pumping session at night, when the body naturally produces more milk.

Many breasts know the difference between Baby and pump, so if you are having a hard time getting enough milk pumped from pumping sessions alone, try pumping on one side while Baby breastfeeds on the other—then switch sides. This way, your baby will trigger the powerful letdown in a way the pump doesn't always do.

Avoid pacifiers and supplementation whenever you are together.

Use a hospital-grade pump.

Drink Fenugreek Tea.

Consider a prescription of Reglan or Domperidone if your supply is dwindling.[37]

Add an extra pumping session to your schedule.

Your state of mind plays a significant role in how much milk you will release. Take a few cleansing, meditative breaths before beginning. Try massaging your breasts for a few minutes before you start. Also be sure to have plenty of water to drink. Yes, I'm talking about wooing yourself so you will put out.

Try, whenever possible, to feed your baby milk you pumped during the day in the daytime and milk you pumped at night in the nighttime. The milk you produce at various times during the 24-hour cycle is tailored specifically to Baby's needs during this time. For example, as we previously learned, milk produced at night is specially tailored to induce sleep.

Altogether

Bottle-feeding can never provide your baby with all the benefits of breastfeeding, but there are some steps you can take to give your baby some significant benefits that many bottle-fed babies do not enjoy. Feed your baby on cue, position the bottle as a breast, partake in plenty of skin-to-skin contact, and remain in close proximity, and you and your baby can enjoy some intimate bonding time as a part of infant feeding.

7

BOOBY BITER

The shockwave of pain that runs through your body is only matched by the paralyzing panic of frantically trying to remove the piranha from your nipple. Biting while breastfeeding can occur with or without teeth, but know that your baby's entry into the world of chompers doesn't have to mean chomping or weaning. Here's the 411 on how to handle your booby biter as you handle all of your parenting challenges: with respect, compassion, and Sage Parenting[19] know-how.

Teethers

If your baby is teething, the urge to bite down is powerful, so a firm "No biting" does not address the underlying need. Instead of fighting against your little one, work with them by *providing them with teethers right before nursing* (frozen bananas, blueberries, and mini bagels are great options for babies older than 6 months, while a wet frozen cloth and toy teethers are best for younger babes). This can satisfy and release the jaw's aggressive energy before that achy, teething mouth takes in your precious nipple.

Exit

The most popular time for biting is at the end of a feeding, when your baby's focus wanes from the serious work of eating and meanders to other things. Try to *be aware of the signs indicating that Baby has finished their main course,* and offer a teether and/or keep your finger right next to Baby's mouth in case they start to bite down. Since babies nurse for a myriad of beneficial reasons beyond hunger, I never removed my baby immediately following his main course, but I learned his cues signaling that his attention had moved on and was at the ready with a knuckle and something he could bite.

Entrance

Feeding your baby on cue, as opposed to attempting to force your little one to breastfeed on your schedule, can also go a long way in setting you both up for success. If they are in an active state and you are trying to impose your agenda against their will, you are asking for trouble. We've all been there. One of the great things about breastfeeding is that it can serve so many purposes: silencer, pacifier, etc. But if Baby is in a biting phase, you must be especially mindful of their state and needs, following their cues for breastfeeding versus chewing. Remember that as your child grows, they earn greater autonomy, including within the breastfeeding relationship.

Cups

It is common for biting to begin around the time the sippy cup enters Baby's world. Some sippy cups have a nipple-like spout that Baby safely chomps as they drink. Then, when Baby is drinking at the breast, they simply continue this learned motion. This one is huge: *Avoid sippy cups with spouts that come anywhere near resembling a nipple* to avoid this problem. A cup with a straw-like apparatus (or even simply giving Baby drinks from an open cup) is a much better option if your baby has this nipple confusion.

Push

Most of us instinctually pull Baby back away from the breast when bitten. This causes Baby to bite down even harder in an attempt to prevent the nipple from slipping out. The last thing you want is to find yourself in a tug-of-war with a little cannibal with your nipple as the prize. Instead, train yourself to react by doing the opposite: *push Baby's face into your breast.* This will make it harder for your baby to breathe through their nose (bear with me for a second) and they will drop open their mouth to take a breath. Again, pushing in leads them to open, pulling away leads them to clamp. You can also wedge your finger in between their gums to lever their mouth the rest of the way open, just enough to retrieve your lost body part.

Response

Babies, especially as they grow older, are little scientists who will repeat behaviors that elicit interesting responses. So your response to being bitten will play an integral role in either indirectly encouraging or extinguishing this behavior. If you react wildly, they will think, "Whoa! What was that? Again!" Whereas a loud yelp and flash of rage could traumatize your baby (Baby jumps and then cries) and can even elicit a nursing strike. A simple but firm, "*Ouch, no bite*" is the best verbal response. You can then offer the breast again. If Baby bites once more, respond again with, "Ouch, no bite," but this time you put the breast away and redirect to another activity. If Baby requests milk again, go through the same process on the other side.

Moving On

As with any parenting challenge that leaves you feeling hurt, it is important to remember that after only a few minutes, Baby has completely moved on. Holding on to any resentment and anger that can grow from hurt will not serve you, your baby, or your relationship. The best thing you can do is address the incident appropriately in the moment so you can both feel resolution and then *let it go.*

Altogether

When my current nursling was around 18 months old, he would bite only when he was transitioning into a deep sleep. His jaw would start to quiver and would then clamp shut (as if forgetting why it was open). So as soon as I felt the quiver, I would quickly put my finger in the corner of his mouth between his gums, break the latch, and separate us.

Biting can be painful, but you can overcome this challenge by offering "yes" biting opportunities, being acutely aware of your baby's state, feeding on cue, avoiding chewable fake nipples, and rewriting your response. Resisting the urge to pull away and instead pushing toward, containing an explosive reaction in favor of a muted but direct, "Ouch, no bite," and then genuinely letting it go all serve to deter biting in a way that leaves your bond intact. Biting, well . . . bites. But as with most parenting challenges, you can combine your innate wisdom and intimate knowledge of your baby with some well-informed strategies to survive and thrive with your baby as a Sage Parent[19].

8

NIGHT WEANING

Many breastfed toddlers reach a point when they figure out that during the day, they do not want to stop being active and having fun to breastfeed. Walking and eating new solid foods are novel skills they are just too excited about to take a break, be still, and nurse. They want to spend the whole day walking, playing, and chowing down on solid food. But they are not yet ready to wean; they still crave the nutrition from breastmilk and the bonding time from breastfeeding. Your toddler is so smart that they may realize that nighttime is boring and the perfect time to make up all that breastfeeding they have cut out of the day.

The long process of your child growing and maturing into their independence is one that they should lead. This should be extended to all aspects of parenting, including breastfeeding. However, I also understand that some people, under certain circumstances, must wean their little one at nighttime in order to get the sleep they need to be a good parent to that child. If you feel that this is the right choice for you and your baby, I can offer you a strategy for night weaning that maintains the dignity, respect, empathy, and compassion with which you parent. This strategy contains no CIO (Cry-It-Out) and does not deny your child you, your comfort, your contact, or your love.

Readiness

Until your little one is old enough to understand what "night-night" means, they are too young for nighttime weaning. Your baby should certainly be at least 12 months old, older if you feel they don't yet have a firm grasp on this concept (ideally 18-24 months). I also want to be clear that this is not a strategy for weaning from breastfeeding in general or an implication, in any way, that babies should be night weaning at 12 months old. If you are happily and functionally night nursing your sweet babe, then embrace it and treasure the time, as it won't last forever, and you will look back on this precious time fondly.

Night-Night

The first step is to introduce your child to the concept of things going night-night. Take some time to begin pointing out all of the things and people around you going night-night like the sun, Daddy, the family pet, etc. Allow this concept to really sink in for a couple weeks. Play this concept out with your child, as play is the learning language of all children. Role-play, use toys, read books, explore nature after dark and your child will understand this concept through positive, fun, educational interaction.

Bedtime Routine

You want to begin your nighttime with a nighttime routine that will help your baby to unwind, calm down, and relax while filling their love cup. I suggest something like saying good-night to the sun and hello to the moon and stars, bath, book (Nursies When the Sun Shines is the perfect companion for my night weaning method), massage, and breastfeeding, as was previously discussed. Infant massage is really the perfect thing to include in your nighttime routine because, in addition to research showing that your baby can sleep longer after a massage, it addresses/prevents a lot of the causes of night waking. You can pick up the Soothing Slumber[33] video to learn this valuable addition to what you can offer your child in easing this transition. A nighttime routine rooted in connection is imperative for this process.

Associations

As you begin this transition, by pointing out that at night the world is sleeping and by setting up a good nighttime routine, also begin to build a sleep cue association. As you breastfeed your little one to sleep, introduce another cue for sleep alongside nursing. For example, softly sing a specific lullaby as you breastfeed them to sleep each night. Perhaps your little one responds well to running your fingers through their hair. Choose something to pair with nursing to sleep so that your child begins to associate all those warm, safe feelings elicited from breastfeeding with your new or additional sleep cue. Then, once the nighttime nursing is gradually removed, you have other comfort options that will be familiar and soothing.

Teddy

Some children have transitional objects like a teddy bear or a baby blanket. My Sky had his "silky B." He needed only walk across it as it lay on the floor and he would collapse into a blissful, cuddly heap. My Bay never had one . . . until he naturally weaned. It is common for children who have used their Mommy Milk as their primary comfort sanctuary (as well they should) to substitute with a comforting object. For Bay, who was infatuated with Peter Pan, his Peter Pan stuffed guy became his new nighttime best friend. As you are pushing this transition before it naturally evolves on its own, it can be helpful to provide options for potential transitional objects that your little one could gravitate toward. So as you move through your nighttime routine, add a little company in the form of a few of their favorite soft lovies.

Window

After you have laid the groundwork with the initial phases of the transition, it is time to set a time window when "milk is night-night." You want to tell your little one during the breastfeeding portion of their nighttime routine that just like sun goes night-night and "Baby" (insert child's name) is going night-night and Mommy is going night-night, "milk" is going to go night-night. Substitute the word "milk" with whatever word you use for breastfeeding. Set aside a brief window of time to start with when the "milk" will be night-night. "Milk" can wake up at sunrise. Since little ones can't tell time, the sun is the perfect indicator for them. For example, if you begin with a window of 4-6 a.m., you breastfeed them each time they wake until 4 a.m. At the last feeding before 4 a.m. you tell your child, "Okay, milk is going night-night. Night-night milk." When the sun wakes up, the milk wakes up. Then if they wake to breastfeed during the 4-6 a.m. window, remind them, "Milk is night-night. When the sun wakes up, the milk wakes up."

Once your baby becomes relatively comfortable with the brief window, you can then expand that window as you desire. Move to 3-6 a.m., then 2-6 a.m., then 1-6 a.m., etc. I advise parents to ultimately land on the hours that the parent sleeps. For example, if you go to sleep at midnight, the "milk" can be night-night from midnight until sunrise. If you say "milk is night-night" and then they cry and you give them milk, it will be a much longer process with more stress and lots of tears. It is important to be consistent; that is why I advise beginning with only a very brief window of time and expanding from there.

For many, a better window is the first stretch of sleep, as they naturally sleep longer during the first portion of the night. In this case, milkies might be night-night if and when Baby wakes before midnight. My go-to starting point in Sage Sleep Email Coaching[80] is actually to have milkies be night-night for the first awakening. Give them the experience of falling asleep without milkies (and with all the alternate sleep cues). Then when they next wake, nurse as usual. The following night, milkies are asleep for the first two awakenings. Continue in this pattern until your babe is night weaned, or until you reach the desired amount of night nursing. This strategy follows a little one's natural sleep rhythm best because they typically sleep longer and deeper the first half of the night and need to nurse frequently and sleep lighter the second half of the night.

Comfort

During this time, your baby will probably be upset, and you are free to follow your maternal instincts and comfort, hold, cuddle, and love them. Your baby is never denied access to the caregivers who love them. Be sure to wear clothing that securely covers your breasts. I know my nursing ninjas could locate, retrieve, and latch a nipple before I even knew what hit me. Keep your breasts out of sight and locked down during this window. Sleeping topless would be like cuddling a cake while you try to kick carbs. Stick with your nighttime boundaries (keep the lights low, stay in your bedroom, etc.), which can provide familiar comfort, offer all those sleep associations and transitional objects you have been building up, and most of all, be a calm, loving, empathetic presence. Be the state you want to see in your baby, and communicate a compassionate confidence. If you trust that your little one will be okay, they will believe it, and they will.

Re-Latch

If you are attempting to wean a younger one, upon upset, re-latch and nurse down to almost asleep, then unlatch again (it can be helpful to press up under the chin to calm the rooting reflex). If they again get upset, nurse down again to almost asleep, then unlatch. Repeat. This will result in less sleep in the short term, but more sleep in the long run as your baby will be learning to fall asleep without the nipple in their mouth.

Altogether

Sleep is one of those things that you have to accept will be different when you make the decision to have a baby. If, after years of meeting your baby's nighttime needs, you feel your child is ready to transition away from nighttime as mealtime, this gentle strategy can facilitate that transition in a way that is loving and comforting and does not rely on isolation or ignoring any of your baby's cues. Using a strategy that allows you to be there and responding sensitively to any distress your baby has during this transition will extend the foundation of trust you have worked so hard to build and provide you both with more sleep.

9

BABY-LED FEEDING

Planning when, how, and what to feed your growing baby can be fun and confusing. There are so many varying opinions, and as with so many things, pop culture takes time to catch up to more informed recommendations. Rest assured that your baby will get the food they need, when they need it, in the way that is best for them to eat it. Baby-led feeding is a natural, stress-free approach to feeding that respects your child and honors their development.

When

A baby should not be exposed to solid foods (anything other than breastmilk) prior to 6 months of age. The previous recommendation from the American Academy of Pediatrics (AAP) was 4-6 months, but we now know that it is in the best interest of babies to wait until the age of 6 months, so the AAP changed their recommendation accordingly.[14] The World Health Organization (WHO), UNICEF, American Academy of Family Physicians, Australian National Health and Medical Research Council, and Health Canada all recommend nothing but breastmilk for the first 6 months of life. Unfortunately, it can take a significant amount of time for a gain in knowledge and change in procedure to trickle down to common knowledge. This fact, along with a completely disproven yet pervasive myth that feeding your baby solid, heavy food will result in more nighttime sleep, results in a lot of pressure on parents to start solids prematurely. Your baby is receiving everything they need from your breastmilk; relax and trust in this perfectly designed infant feeding system. Once your baby hits the 6-months mark, you can look for cues of developmental interest in eating and offer them food. Staring at your food going from your plate to your mouth, reaching for the spoon or fork, and mimic chewing can all be signs that your baby is ready to be exposed to the real thing.

What

Question conventional tradition when it comes to what to feed your baby for his first meals. Seek nutritional information and consider your family's food culture along with any food issues specific to your baby. Research has taught us that there is no one right answer when it comes to what to feed your baby. Indian families tend to feed their babies spicier, flavor-rich foods, and they have the same positive outcomes as families who take a more American, bland foods first approach. If you wouldn't consider a white rice cereal the healthiest option for you, then choose a healthier option for your baby. You are both the same species; you can offer your baby some of the food you are eating. Just be mindful of bite size, texture, and consistency to avoid choking.

Rice cereal has long been given to American babies as a first food. However, it can lead to obesity, cause constipation, and lacks nutrients. There is never a reason to add rice cereal to a bottle, which some mistakenly believe will result in more sleep at night. This is a disproven myth. It actually results in less sleep because it causes gastrointestinal distress while providing none of the nutrition the breastmilk would have provided, so Baby is bothered by an upset stomach and craving nutrition sooner. Other disproven myths include rice cereal curing acid reflux or resolving spitting up.[39] Think instead about foods that are in your family's diet that would be fun and healthy for your little one to explore. Some of my favorites are foods such as avocados, bananas, and carrots.

How

Eating begins as a development exercise in fine motor control, hand-eye coordination, behavior modeling ("eating like mommy"), exploring textures and tastes, etc. You don't need to "feed" your baby. Instead "offer" or "serve" your baby food. There is no pressing need to shovel spoonfuls of food in their mouth against their will. Your child's relationship with eating begins with you providing the developmental opportunity for your child to mimic your eating behaviors. Allow your baby to play with a baby spoon and bowl while you eat. Put a small serving of food in front of your baby and allow them to explore it. Your baby will mush it in between their fingers, lick it, smear it, smell it, explore the texture, etc. There is no need to get a certain amount of food in your baby's stomach. Your baby wants to practice mimicking your eating behavior while exploring food. It is a developmental exercise that, if allowed to take place, can start your child down a path of healthful eating habits. Continue offering your baby food, and as they become more competent and hungry, they will get and want more and more food in their mouth. It should be positive and fun with an emphasis on exploration.

West's first food was avocado. We were eating food with avocado, and after he was lunging for our plates, staring at our mouths, and pretending to chew (and he had hit the 6-months mark), I mashed some up and put it in front of him. He wasn't a big fan of the avocado itself, but he thoroughly enjoyed being included, and his eyes were wild with excitement over the new experience of being given the opportunity to "eat" (as in the behaviors of meal time). Shortly thereafter I was eating a banana and he went after it. I allowed him to hold it and gnaw on the banana. He *loved* it. I was careful to watch every gum mark and inventory the banana itself to keep an eye out for any chunks that he might have gnawed off, but he just sucked and gummed while excitedly practicing all those eating behaviors and working on the fine motor skills required for eating. It was great, and we have all had an easy, fun time with the process of introducing our youngest to the wild world of delicious foods!

The tradition of shoveling spoonfuls of white mush into your baby's mouth at 4 months old as a rite of passage has been overhauled. Wait until 6 months of age, offer your baby a food that you deem appropriate, and allow your baby to explore the behavior of eating from a developmental and experiential perspective.

10

MASTER MEALTIME

You're on a natural parenting path and you want to extend that wholesome, nutritive start that breastfeeding has provided. You are choosing what goes into your bodies with great intention, serving organic gluten-, sugar-, and artificial dye-free veg grown in a field grazed by unicorns (who fertilize the soil with rainbows) that is harvested by a circle of doula fairies singing "Imagine" (the Eva Cassidy version, of course). Or maybe not. But the parenting side of eating can often prove more challenging than we realize, as the weight of our own baggage around eating can prove heavy to bear.

Mainstream Approach

Control

"You must clean your plate before you may be excused."

"If you're good, you can have some dessert."

We are all born with the innate ability to listen to our bodies. If nothing else, a baby knows when they are hungry. As children get older, parents (and other sources) can interfere with this communication between brain and body. "Clean your plate. We worked hard to make this dinner for you. You cannot get down from this table until you eat every bite." *It is your job as a parent to provide your child with healthy food. It is not your job to make them eat it.* If and how much they eat is up to them, with encouragement from you to listen to the cues of their body.

When you force a child to eat, you teach them to ignore the signals of hunger and fullness they receive from their body. When you respect what your child tells you about their eating, you are teaching them to listen to and respect what their body is telling them. Giving them the control of what goes into their body and allowing them to suffer the natural consequences of not listening to their body's cues will remove the power struggle between you and eliminate issues surrounding emotional eating. A child who is provided healthy food but not forced to eat will not associate food with a loss of control or emotions such as guilt or approval.

Reward/Punishment

You know better than to use rewards and punishments (because you have read the Sage Parenting book[19], where you learned why they suck and how they don't work). Food is an especially dangerous area to enact this parenting tactic of control, so it's worth addressing. Using food as a reward and/or punishment is a surefire way to raise an emotional eater. A child who is consistently rewarded with unhealthy foods builds a lifelong association between unhealthy food and feelings of approval and acceptance. It's a simple case of conditioning. Achievement is met with a pleasing expression of approval, and feelings of pride, love, and self-confidence—with dessert. Eventually you can remove the achievement and elicit those positive feelings with only the dessert. As an adult you find yourself coping with experiences that starve your sense of approval, love, and self-confidence by eating dessert, which has been conditioned to nourish those same feelings. A child who has food withheld to communicate a sense of disapproval and disappointment can have issues of control and overeating, giving themselves lots of food to overcome those feelings when they experience them as an adult. An occasional trip to the ice cream store with the baseball team after a win or removing the dinner plate of a child who is throwing their food is fine. Consistently using food as a disciplinary tool will not yield the desired result of a healthy, happy, well-adjusted adult.

Altogether

"Two nutritionists in Illinois conducted a fascinating experiment a few years ago. They observed 77 children between the ages of two and four, and also learned how much their parents attempted to control their eating habits. They discovered that those parents who insisted their children eat only during mealtimes (rather than when they were hungry), or who encouraged them to clean their plates (even when they obviously weren't hungry), or who used food (especially desserts) as a reward, wound up with children who lost the ability to regulate their caloric intake. Some of the parents appeared to have their own issues with food, which were in the process of passing on to their kids. But whatever the reason for their excessive control, it was beginning to take its toll even before some of these children were out of diapers. The children had 'few opportunities to learn to control their own food intake' and came to stop trusting their bodies' cues about when they were hungry. One result: Many of them were already starting to get fat."[15]

Natural Eating

Grazing

Now that we've taken a small detour through where you don't want to go, let's get back on our Sage Parenting path. You know how beautifully breastfeeding on cue has met your baby's needs and fostered a strong brain-body connection? Let's extend that same path beyond the breast to eating on cue. When trusted and honored, little ones fall into a natural pattern of eating referred to as grazing. Instead of sitting down to three large meals, they, with their small stomachs and high-energy needs, seek frequent, small snacks on the go. Basically, they listen to the needs of their bodies and eat when hungry, stopping when not. This style of consuming calories is to be encouraged, as it truly is what they need at this stage of the eating game. The older your child becomes, the more they will eat during meals and the less they will need those frequent snacks. (Though it is actually healthier even for an adult to eat numerous small meals or healthy snacks throughout the day than a few large meals, so you can ditch the judgment piece).

Accessibility

Keeping quality foods readily available and accessible can support this healthy and natural eating behavior. For us, this looks like having prepped and child portioned foods in the bottom pantry and fridge drawers. From a very young age my children are able to meet their own needs (independence) using the internal cues of their bodies as a guide. As they grow, they are welcome with me or their daddy in the kitchen, and then on their own. As I write this, my 8-year-old is excitedly making some food for us all in the kitchen, and last night my 11-year-old made us all a delicious soup. The opposite of this would look like children who are only allowed to eat what they are served. I sometimes hear parents say, "Oh I could never do that. My children would eat everything!" I have to ask, "Then what happens when they are on their own?" Choose what you bring into your home with intention and grant your children free access. If you trust them from the beginning, they will benefit from self-regulation for the long haul.

Offer

A staple shift from the mainstream approach most of us endured as children is to *offer, not feed*. The best place to start is actually with your language. "I'm making some scrambled eggs. Would you like some?" will support the respectful relationship you seek better than turning to your partner and saying, "I'm going to feed him." This can also be a huge weight lifted for most of us (parents and children alike). Provide good foods and invite them into the eating world, then respect their choices. Trust them—it will all work out.

Environment

Creating a child-sized eating environment is one way to extend that invitation (size down). Providing your young child with a booster seat and child-sized utensils can go a long way in making them feel comfortable at mealtime. If you want your child to feel included and be successful with mealtime behavior, then they can't feel like they don't fit. Using a booster seat (or your lap) means that your child will have an equal seat at the table and be at the appropriate eating height. A young person, working hard on perfecting their fine motor skills, will not be very successful at getting an appropriately sized bite of food on the fork and in their mouth with a heavy fork that is too deep to go all the way in their mouth. The simple step of placing a child-sized fork at their place setting will go a long way in setting them up for success with mealtime coordination and manners.

Portion

Your child needs a much smaller portion size than an adult. This is where having a child-sized plate or bowl comes in handy. When serving food, we tend to gear the portion size to the dish, not the person. Your child's stomach is a fraction of the size of yours. Placing a mountain of food in front of them implies that you expect them to eat that much food. You don't want to inadvertently pressure your child to eat more than their body is telling them they need. A big plate with an adult-sized serving of food can also be overwhelming for a child. Imagine if you worked in an office and your boss walked up to your desk and dropped a giant stack of paperwork right in front of you. How would that make you feel? Initially serve your child only a small portion. If they ask for more when they're finished, you can always give them more.

Balanced Diet

One way to start this off on the right foot is to use a sectioned plate. A plate with small sections will set you up to provide a small volume of food from the different food groups: a fruit, veggie, grain, protein and dairy. If you only provide, say, two of the food groups, the other empty sections are staring right at you. It makes it pretty darn foolproof to provide well-balanced meals

for your children. The same is true for to-go snacks (for which a bento box is great). Filling them themselves provides them with a great sense of autonomy and personal responsibility while instilling in them an understanding of healthy eating habits—all while being super easy for us as parents. Today, for example, I believe Bay took turkey, crackers, cheese, and grapes, and he always has water with him. When preparing meals, be sure to include at least one thing your child likes, but then you can include some other things they may just taste or be exposed to. Though, if you've been on this path from the beginning, you really can trust that the nutrition piece will work out as it needs to for your child today. Some days that might look like vegetable and fruit smoothies all day. Still other days it might look like pasta with a side of pasta. Children go through big developmental and physical growth spurts in which they sometimes crave unique things. Honoring the cues of their body is the key and you want to support that. As they get older, you can further parse this down with "tongue or tummy"? "My taste buds have a hankering for a cookie right now but my body is actually hungry for some protein.
Hmmmm . . ." Invite your children into those honest inner dialogues and they will learn to identify and weigh their choices in the same way.

Kitchen

Looking at the broader environmental picture, you want to make a healthy and accessible kitchen. If you fill your kitchen with healthy foods, then that is what your family has to choose from. If you open your pantry and see unhealthy options, then that is what you will eat and your children will want. When you go grocery shopping, make a list with your child (you can even make a separate list for your child with pictures so they can help), be sure to shop when you are not hungry (I am so guilty of this), and organize your food in such a way that healthy food is convenient and accessible. One simple example of this is a fruit bowl that sits on the counter. See the apple, grab it, and go! The other piece to an ideal culinary environment is that your child needs access to the kitchen. If they want to wash dishes, let them. If they want to cut fruit, give them a banana and a butter knife. Experience builds competence.

Spirit

Is mealtime a time of positive connection? Is your kitchen a canvas of exploration and inclusion? Do you continue to be open and flexible even when the mainstream mealtime pressures of manners and rigidity creep into your consciousness? Are you able to tap into your sense of humor and let messes happen for the sake of learning, experience, and independence? One of our kids' favorite mealtime activities is to go around the table and all answer one question. For example, "How were you brave today?"; "How did you fail today?"; "How were you kind today?"; "What is something you appreciate about each person?"; "What was your sweetest memory of the day?"; or "What was your biggest challenge today?" Most importantly, create the spirit of mealtime with intention. Remove any and all pressure and don't feel a need to even speak about the food at all. Mealtime is an opportunity for connection. The food is secondary.

Shifting that focus will release any pressure. Remember, you're just offering (and are not concerned with whether or how much they eat). You won't just be telling your kids to eat healthily—you will be living a lifestyle integrated with healthy eating habits.

Altogether

"I need help getting my son to eat. Mealtimes are a nightmare that leaves me beyond frustrated. I work so hard to cook him good food, and no matter what I do he just won't eat like he should, and he just wants to get down and leave. I want him to be a good eater. And I never get to eat in all this back and forth."

What is a good eater? Where does your idea of what your child "should" eat like come from? What would a peaceful mealtime look like? What are *your* mealtime needs? Let's redefine. You don't have control (or responsibility) over how much they eat. Let that sink in for a minute. You cannot will your child to be any way they are not (or not be a way they are). Your deep investment in how much they eat will only serve to drive them away from healthy eating, create issues of control around food for them for life, and leave you feeling like a failure every mealtime. We can set a boundary for self-care. So how do we make this shift? You are going to let go of your attachment to how much they eat completely. Now, while you cannot control how much they eat,, you can control what foods are offered and the spirit of mealtime. So here's what this will look like:

- You will make a meal that includes small portions of a variety of foods (balanced diet). One of the items on their plate should always be something you know they crave right now (something they will definitely like and eat).

- You will not say anything related to their food consumption during mealtime. (No wonder they want to run away if they are being cajoled the whole time they are sitting at the table, right?). Talk about your day. Share a sweet memory. Conversation—no food talk.

- They are free to leave the table and come and go. Their plate remains on the table until bedtime. If they express hunger anytime after dinner, you can remind them that they are welcome to eat their dinner, which is on the table. If they express dissatisfaction with what food is before them, you will tell yourself, "This is not a rejection of my efforts. This is not an unwillingness to be the child I want them to be. This is just a preference. I will hear it. I will validate it. 'You want sausage for dinner tonight. We are having pasta. You are disappointed by that.'"

- When you sit down to eat, you will set a timer. When that timer dings, you can get down from the table and join them upon request. But until that timer (which they can see and hear ticking) dings, it is Mommy's turn to eat. Anytime they cry for you to come, I want you say to yourself, "I am wanted." And say to them once, "When the timer dings, Mommy's turn to eat is all done and I will join you. You are welcome to sit with me here while I eat." Once this is established, the timer will no longer be necessary. You will be free to honor your body's cues, being a wonderful role model for your child.

11

THE BREAST SEASON

You're all too willing to spend hours cuddled up nursing in the mornings, preparing for the drought from distraction the day brings. I sense that you feel the coming change of seasons too, as the milk seems to taste that much more sweet to you and these moments that much more precious.

Your small hand resting lovingly on my chest is no longer a passive recipient of my loving touch. It now creeps across me with its own priorities that amuse and distract us both.

I could stay lost in this connection with you all day, but I know we won't. Like a small thorn in the bands of love that bind us, my bliss is pricked by the thought that this will end.

In this most holy of pockets of energy in the universe, I am united with the millions of other maternal goddesses who are nourishing and defining humanity with health and love through this act.

As a nursing session ends with your desire to otherwise conquer the world, the euphoric drunkenness of our oxytocin time-out fades and I am left with empty arms. They are strong arms that defend and build and hug, but their strength was forged under the weight of you and your brothers, and the ache of my gratitude is always present in their use.

My fingers delicately touch the top of my breast to feel the ghost of your hand while my body and mind have moved forward in sync with you in the present. The warmth of my fingertips betrays my unconscious mind, staying with my heart just a step behind the moments that are fading.

You bloom remarkably, having surpassed the size and cleverness of most long ago. There is no greater harbinger of pride for a mother than the joyful song that accompanies a blooming bud. But the quiet, dull ache of longing is always there below the surface when one becomes two.

As you skip over to me, giddy for your "Mup!", I collapse in around you, knowing soon you will be skipping over for only a hug.

These are the final months with my final nursling, and I can feel the Earth shifting beneath us, gradually as it always is, but me now acutely aware of the momentum. The changes in my body chemistry spurred by your cheerful insistence to progress on your journey, is heralding the change of seasons. My fertile spring is ending and, as the days warm and the sun shines that much more beautifully and harshly, summer is on the horizon. I never resist— what a futile and counterproductive effort that would be. I merely revel fully in the sweet taste of the present.

The bittersweet acknowledgment of the change of season swirling around my blooming bud makes my heart heavy with warm gratitude for every step on our breastfeeding journey and all this season gifts us for the future.

Weaning

When the sun is setting on your breastfeeding journey, you might be taken by surprise at the profound and significant physiological and emotional effects. Whether initiated by you for a practical reason or gradually unfolded in your child's own time, the transition of weaning is poignant.

Your emotional world will be rocked, and I don't mean like that fly Eric Hutchinson concert I just attended at the beach ("If you wanna rock, you rock...")[76]. You may have felt touched out and ready for autonomy and space, but once breastfeeding has ceased, you may feel as though the emotional floor has dropped—you are mourning. Remember, breastfeeding bathes your brain in mood-boosting feel-good hormones like oxytocin: nature's postpartum antidepressant. Awareness of this phenomenon can help you to overcome it. Know that whatever out of character thoughts, feelings, or apathy you are experiencing are likely the weaning talking. So don't make any big life decisions or changes while under the influence of the short-lived weaning depression (an area of study that is in desperate need of researching). Shore up your support systems at the start of the transition, before you are in the thick of it and potentially in an unclear fog. For me, that looks like explaining what could potentially be expected with my husband so he would know to be extra gentle with my feelings and extra helpful in picking up any slack. I would stock my kitchen with foods that make me feel good. I would reach out to my close friends and plan outdoor play dates to keep me connected with nature (vitamin D from the sunshine helps) and the world.

Also, stay in touch with your body, as your breasts might need a more gradual transition than your child prefers. To avoid discomforts such as mastitis and plugged ducts, you may need to express milk just for a little while, tapering down. Someone with a strong supply, whose little one nursed three times a day and has now ceased altogether, may need to hand express or pump twice a day, then once, then be done. A fun tip is to freeze that final breastmilk so you still have some on hand for things like ear infections or rashes. Though with child-led weaning, this is rarely necessary. The good news is that this period is short-lived, and after your chemistry adjusts to the absence of the extra oxytocin, the vast majority of women return to normal, in a new homeostasis, feeling balanced and like themselves again. If these feelings don't fade and the depression persists or worsens to the point of significant struggle, I definitely recommend seeing a quality marital and family therapist (MFT) who can help.

One special tool in easing through this transition is ritual to honor your breastfeeding journey. I ordered myself a breastmilk pendant necklace that I will treasure forever (a gift to myself). You can write a letter to your child. I love the idea of creating a picture book of special breastfeeding memories. Some have parties while others share a special day with their child to celebrate the change in the relationship. Choose something that feels right for you and your little one and honor the shit out of this amazing gift you have given your child.

After 10 years of breastfeeding three little ones, this season is ending for me, and I'm feeling all the feels. My breasts feel quiet, relaxed, and proud while my heart feels a bit raw, yet full. My youngest just turned 5, and his last nursing sessions when waking are the exception rather than the rule. We have chosen to let it fade naturally and quietly. He's cuddling alongside me right now as I type this, and he gives me spontaneous kisses while I stroke his hair. The connection doesn't go away, it changes form. My three boys may no longer spend their days cuddled on my chest nursing but they do spend their days adventuring, learning, growing, and thriving in connection with each other, their daddy, and me (more on this in the Sage Homeschooling book[81]). I'm choosing to hold gratitude and reverence for my body as I move into this new season of life where my value is no longer rooted in my youth or fertility. I stand tall in my beautiful feminine stature, with a strong marriage and three shining young men, having no regrets for any of the time or energy I poured into nourishing my children over the last decade. I find us standing in a place of independence, health, and love, and that was all forged in the milky fire of our breastfeeding relationship.

It was easy. It was hard. It was beautiful. It was messy. It was peaceful. It was chaotic. It WAS. That is worth honoring.

THE NEXT STEP

Welcome to the Sage Parenting family!

Coaching

You've read the guidebook for walking the Sage Breastfeeding path; it's a journey that is endlessly fulfilling and rarely perfect. That's why I offer one-on-one coaching. This guidebook can take you so far, but sometimes you just need a personalized guide in your pocket (that's me—it's cozier in here than you might think). Every little one is unique, so sometimes a general theme won't fit without the customized piece to translate it into your child's natural language. I'm here. I see you. I can help, with small shifts that yield huge results. And because you are now in the club, you get to enjoy 10% off your first coaching package with the code LOYALSAGE.

Books

Feeding is one trail on the Sage Parenting path. Sleep, homeschooling and parenting are also important trails on the Sage Parenting path. So important, in fact, that they have their own guidebooks. Sage Breastfeeding is book three in a four-part series. Walk deeper down the path with:

Sage Parenting: Honored and Connected
Sage Sleep: Rested and Connected
Sage Homeschooling: Wise and Connected

References

1. Balancing Breastfeeding by Danelle Frisbie: http://www.drmomma.org/2010/01/balancing-breastfeeding-when-moms-must.html
2. Breastfeeding by the World Health Organization: http://www.who.int/topics/breastfeeding/en/
3. AAP Reaffirms Breastfeeding Guidelines by the American Academy of Pediatrics: http://www.aap.org/en-us/about-the-aap/aap-press-room/pages/AAP-Reaffirms-Breastfeeding-Guidelines.aspx?nfstatus=401&nftoken=00000000-0000-0000-0000-000000000000&nfstatusdescription=ERROR%3a+No+local+token
4. Breastfeeding a Toddler by the International Breastfeeding Centre: http://www.nbci.ca/index.php?option=com_content&view=article&id=78:breastfeed-a-toddlerwhy-on-earth&catid=5:information&Itemid=17
5. WHO Growth Standards are Recommended for Use in the US for Infants and Children 0 to 2 Years of Age by the Centers for Disease Control and Prevention (CDC): http://www.cdc.gov/growthcharts/who_charts.htm
6. How Does Milk Production Work by Kelly Bonyata: http://kellymom.com/pregnancy/bf-prep/milkproduction/
7. How many days will it take for my milk to come in by Jan Barger: http://www.babycenter.com/404_how-many-

days-will-it-take-for-my-milk-to-come-in_8897.bc

8. Supplementing the Breastfeeding Baby by Auerbach, K., Montgomery, A.: http://www.lalecheleague.org/llleaderweb/lv/lvaugsep99p75.html

9. Human Milk 4 Human Babies: https://www.facebook.com/hm4hb

10. The Clash. 1982. Rock the Casbah. *Combat Rock.*

11. How Does Formula Compare to Breastmilk by the California Department of Health Services (WIC): http://www.cdph.ca.gov/programs/breastfeeding/Documents/MO-HowDoesForWAFBF-Eng.pdf

12. Breastfeeding vs. Formula Feeding by Kids Health: http://kidshealth.org/parent/growth/feeding/breast_bottle_feeding.html#

13. Did you ever wonder what's in Breastmilk Versus Formula by Heslett, C., Hedberg, S., Rumble, H.: http://www.bcbabyfriendly.ca/whatsinbreastmilkposter.pdf

14. Breastfeeding Initiatives by the American Academy of Pediatrics (AAP): http://www2.aap.org/breastfeeding/faqsbreastfeeding.html

15. Unconditional Parenting By Alfie Kohn: http://www.unconditionalparenting.com/UP/

16. Family Dinners Are Important by Jeanie Lerche Davis http://children.webmd.com/guide/family-dinners-are-important

17. Terri Westcott Athey, 2012

18. Melatonin, Babies, and Breastmilk by Dr. Sheryl Wagner:

http://drsherylwagner.blogspot.com/2012/10/melatonin-babies-and-breastmilk.html

19. Sage Parenting: Honored and Connected by Rachel Rainbolt: http://www.sageparenting.com/sage-parenting-book

20. Every Argument Against NIP Debunked by Elsinora: http://community.babycenter.com/post/a31512833/every_argument_against_nip_debunked_-_newly_expanded

21. Nursing in Public Discrimination: My Journey by Rachel Rainbolt: http://www.sageparenting.com/nursing-in-public-discrimination

22. California Unruh Complaint of Discrimination: http://www.dfeh.ca.gov

23. Infant Feeding and Childhood Cognition at Ages 3 and 7 years by Belfort, M., et al. (JAMA Pediatrics): http://archpedi.jamanetwork.com/article.aspx?articleid=1720224

24. Breast feeding reduces risk of breast cancer, study says by Isabel Woodman: http://www.ncbi.nlm.nih.gov/pmc/articles/PMC1143616/

25. The Burden of Suboptimal Breastfeeding in the United States by Bartick, M., Reinhold, A. (Pediatrics): http://pediatrics.aappublications.org/content/125/5/e1048.full

26. The Badass Breastfeeder: http://www.thebadassbreastfeeder.com

27. Mary Breastfeeds Jesus:
http://www.huffingtonpost.com/2012/12/11/mary-breastfeeding-jesus_n_2274119.html
28. Victorian Breastfeeding Photos:
http://www.huffingtonpost.com/2013/06/17/victorian-breastfeeding-photo_n_3442872.html
29. No Honey for Infants:
http://www.infantbotulism.org/parent/No_Honey_Brochure_English.pdf
30.   WHO Growth Standards are Recommended for Use in the US for Infants and Children 0 to 2 Years of Age by the Centers for Disease Control and Prevention (CDC):
http://www.cdc.gov/growthcharts/who_charts.htm
31. Covering Up is a Feminist Issue by Annie (PhD in Parenting):
http://www.phdinparenting.com/blog/2010/1/27/covering-up-is-a-feminist-issue.html
32. Breastfeeding Laws:
http://breastfeedinglaw.com/state-laws/california/
33. Booby Traps by Best for Babes:
https://www.bestforbabes.org/what-are-the-booby-traps
34.   Best for Babes:
https://www.bestforbabes.org
35. Gastroesophageal Reflux Disease by Dr. Esther Entin:
http://www.thedoctorwillseeyounow.com/content/kids/art3497.html
36. The Newborn's Stomach by Katie Wickham:
http://babiesfirstlactation.wordpress.com/2013/08/09/the-newborns-stomach/

37. Increasing Your Milk Supply by Anne Smith: http://www.breastfeedingbasics.com/articles/increasing-your-milk-supply
38. Practical Bottle Feeding Tips by Healthy Children http://www.healthychildren.org/English/ages-stages/baby/feeding-nutrition/pages/Practical-Bottle-Feeding-Tips.aspx
39. Skip the Baby Cereal by Breastfeeding Mama Talk: http://www.breastfeedingmamatalk.com/dangers-of-rice-cereal/#.Uz22Htz7Z2G
40.   5 Cool Things No One Ever Told You About Nighttime Breastfeeding by Breastfeed Chicago: http://breastfeedchicago.wordpress.com/2013/05/24/5-cool-things-no-one-ever-told-you-about-nighttime-breastfeeding/
41. Biological Nurturing: http://www.biologicalnurturing.com
42. Mastitis by the Mayo Clinic: http://www.mayoclinic.org/diseases-conditions/mastitis/basics/definition/con-20026633
43.   Foremilk Hindmilk Imbalance by Breastfeeding Problems: http://www.breastfeeding-problems.com/foremilk-hindmilk-imbalance.html
44.   Sage Baby: Baby Massage and Beyond by Rachel Rainbolt: http://www.sageparenting.com/sage-baby-class/
45. Breastfeeding After Breast and Nipple Surgeries: http://www.bfar.org/index.shtml
46.   Tell Me About Tongue Ties! By Norma Ritter:

https://breastfeedingusa.org/content/article/tell-me-about-tongue-ties

47. Dairy and other Food Sensitivites in Breastfed Babies by Kelly Bonyata: http://kellymom.com/health/baby-health/food-sensitivity/

48.   Sage Sleep: Rested and Connected by Rachel Rainbolt: http://www.sageparenting.com/sage-nighttime-parenting-book/

49.   Virtual Breastfeeding Culture by Lara Audelo: http://virtualbreastfeedingculture.com

50.   Daytime Nursing Bra: http://www.bravadodesigns.com/shop/the-body-silk-seamless-nursing-bra

51. Nighttime Nursing Bra: http://www.medela.com/IW/en/breastfeeding/products/intimate-apparel/bras-and-top.html

52. Toddler Tula: http://www.tulababycarriers.com/collections/ergonomic-baby-carrier-toddler

53. Baby K'tan http://www.babyktan.com

54. Moby Wrap: http://www.mobywrap.com/mw/Home.htm

55. Ergo Baby: http://store.ergobaby.com

56. Boppy Breastfeeding Pillow: http://www.boppy.com

57. 5 Things You Thought You Knew About Breastfeeding by Darcia Narvaez: http://www.psychologytoday.com/blog/moral-

landscapes/201108/5-things-you-thought-you-knew-about-breastfeeding

58. Parent Like a Caveman by Danielle Friedman: http://www.thedailybeast.com/articles/2010/10/11/hunter-gatherer-parents-better-than-todays-moms-and-dads.html

59. A New Look at the Safety of Breastfeeding During Pregnancy by Hilary Dervin Flower: http://kellymom.com/pregnancy/bf-preg/bfpregnancy_safety/

60. Breastfeeding and Fertility by Christine Foster: http://www.lalecheleague.org/nb/nbsepoct06p196.html

61. Breast feeding reduces the risk of cancer, says study by Isabel Woodman: http://www.ncbi.nlm.nih.gov/pmc/articles/PMC1143616/

62. Breast Cancer Risk Reduced by 50 Percent by Breastfeeding for 2 or More Years by Yale News: http://news.yale.edu/2001/01/25/breast-cancer-risk-reduced-50-percent-breastfeeding-two-or-more-years

63. Is Breastfeeding Linked to Tooth Decay? By Kelly Bonyata: http://kellymom.com/health/baby-health/tooth-decay/

64. Study Finds No Association Between Breastfeeding and Early Childhood Caries by the American Dental Association: http://www.ada.org/3143.aspx

65. 5 Reasons American Women Won't Breastfeed by Rani Molla: http://blogs.wsj.com/five-things/2014/04/14/5-

reasons-american-women-wont-
breastfeed/?KEYWORDS=breastfeeding

66.   The Ugly Side of Nursing Rooms by Abby
Theuring:
http://www.thebadassbreastfeeder.com/the-
ugly-side-of-nursing-rooms/

67. Jennifer Heisleman Ingalls, RN, MSN, OCN, CNL,
2014

68.   Nursies When the Sun Shines by Katherine
Havener: http://nursiesbook.com

69.   Soothing Slumber by Rachel Rainbolt:
http://www.sageparenting.com/soothing-
slumber-video/

70.   Earth Mama Angel Baby: Natural Nipple
Butter:
http://www.earthmamaangelbaby.com/breastfee
ding-support/natural-nipple-butter.html

71. Breastfeeding and Alcohol Consumption:
http://evolutionaryparenting.com/guest-post-
breastfeeding-and-alcohol-consumption/

72. Pope Francis Urges Moms to Breastfeed:
http://www.huffingtonpost.com/2014/01/13/pope-
francis-breastfeeding_n_4585970.html and
http://www.npr.org/sections/thetwo-
way/2017/01/09/508927895/pope-francis-
reiterates-support-for-public-breastfeeding

73. Medications and Mother's Milk:
http://www.amazon.com/Medications-Mothers-
Milk-Lactational-Pharmacology/dp/096362198X

74. Infant Risk Center:
http://www.infantrisk.com

75. LactMed:
http://toxnet.nlm.nih.gov/help/lactmedapp.htm

76. Eric Hutchinson, Rock and Roll:
http://www.erichutchinson.com/main/

77. Nursing While Babywearing:
https://youtu.be/Y4dojl8Qt7Q

78. Baby's Breastie: http://babysbreastie.com

79. Casey Ebert, 2015

80. Sage Email Coaching:
http://www.sageparenting.com/parenting-
coaching/

81. Sage Homeschooling:
http://www.sageparenting.com/sage-
homeschooling-book/

82. Leptin:
https://www.ncbi.nlm.nih.gov/m/pubmed/169880
79/

Made in United States
North Haven, CT
21 December 2021

13487196R00068